Progress in Cerebrovascular Disease

Progress in Cerebrovascular Disease

Current Concepts in Stroke and Vascular Dementia

Editors

J. S. Chopra
K. Jagannathan
I. M. S. Sawhney
H. Lechner
G. L. Szendey

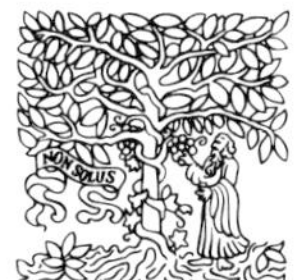

1990

ELSEVIER Amsterdam, New York, Oxford

ISBN 0 444 81421 3

This book is printed on acid-free paper.

Published by:
Elsevier Science Publishers B.V.
(Biomedical Division)
P.O. Box 211
1000 AE Amsterdam
The Netherlands

Sole distributors for the USA and Canada:
Elsevier Science Publishing Company Inc.
655 Avenue of the Americas
New York, NY 10010
USA

This volume has been prepared using the newly developed method of electronic text processing, generally known as Desktop Publishing. In order to ensure rapid publication, while at the same time maintaining the highest degree of scientific accuracy and consistency of style, the manuscripts have only been subjected to basic linguistic editing.

Printed in The Netherlands

Introduction

George L. Szendey
Pharmaceutical Division, Hoechst Aktiengesellschaft, Frankfurt am Main, Germany

Although the incidence of stroke has been reduced in a number of countries as the result of better control of hypertension and other risk factors, there is every prospect that the total number of stroke victims worldwide will rise sharply over the next decades.

Reports from a number of countries clearly show that by the turn of the century many more people will live to an age at which cerebrovascular disease is a common occurrence. According to these sources, rising living standards and the conquest of many formerly rampant diseases, especially in the developing world with its young populations, will greatly increase life expectancy. A rise in cerebrovascular disease will be the inevitable result of this development.

Part One of this volume compiles the papers of the session on Acute Cerebrovascular Disease.

Neuroepidemiological studies indicate that transient ischaemic attacks, hypertension, myocardial ischaemic diseases, diabetes and smoking habits are major predicting risk factors for ischaemic stroke, as summarized by B.P.M. Schulte, The Netherlands.

Ischaemic stroke as the most severe manifestation of acute cerebrovascular disease is caused by either thrombosis due to atherosclerosis including emboli from carotid artery plaques, embolic strokes of cardiac origin and lacunar strokes due to arteriolar occlusion or cerebral microangiopathies. The latter includes the impairment of blood flow properties due to pathological changes in haemorheological parameters, particularly in the cerebral microcirculation.

A critical factor in acute cerebrovascular accidents is very often constituted by platelet adhesion on the basis of platelet aggregation and endothelial damage.

K. Kogure, Japan, suggests that sudden cerebral arterial occlusions leading to acute and chronic brain cell damage are characterized by neuronal mechanisms such as energy failure and loss of both structural and functional integrity of the cell membrane.

Acute cerebral ischaemia affects the functional cellular metabolism in the ischaemic territory. At the center of the infarction, tissue damage may occur but in the so-called penumbra, cell integrity may be preserved if reduction of tissue perfusion does not exceed a threshold value. A critical evaluation of the role of haemodilution as well as of haemorheological factors is presented by A. Hartmann, Germany.

J.S. Chopra, India, reports on acute cerebral venous occlusions, a fairly fatal condition common in India among child-bearing women or women who have just given birth. Curiously enough, all the women suffering venous stroke have had their confinements at home where – for traditional reasons – they have been deprived of water for one or two days. This suggests a possible relationship between the steep increase in blood viscosity and cerebral venous thrombosis.

Transient ischaemic attacks (TIA), often ignored by the patient, are increasingly recognized as precursors of serious cerebrovascular events. J.F. Toole, USA, argues that the arbitrary definition of TIA was established at a time when advanced diagnostic techniques such as CAT scan or MRI were unknown. The return of the function of briefly impaired areas after TIA does not mean that there is no permanent brain damage. About 36% of the patients have an infarction within the month and 50% within 12 months after the onset of TIA.

Stroke in the young is a frequent problem in the host country of the XIVth WCN, India. Hypertension, dyslipidaemia, high haematocrits, vasculitis and the use of oestrogenes are named by P.M. Dalal, India, as predominant causes of stroke in people aged 11 to 45.

Acute ischaemic stroke therapy is discussed by F.M. Yatsu, USA. Therapeutic measures are directed towards the thrombus, to the improvement of collateral circulation, particularly in the 'ischaemic penumbra', and to the prevention of secondary metabolic events, resulting from ischaemia and reperfusion which can aggravate the cerebral insult in precipitating irreversible neuronal damage.

Part Two of this volume presents the current concepts of Chronic Cerebrovascular Disease.

Vascular dementia (VD) is one of the most common forms of chronic cerebrovascular disease. It is currently considered as a severely frequent cause of dementia after the senile dementia of Alzheimer type (DAT).

Carlo Loeb of Italy claims that the term vascular dementia seems more appropriate to identify conditions of intellectual impairment due to vascular origin than the term multi-infarct dementia (MID).

The clinical diagnosis should include the identification of the dementia syndrome (history, neurological examination, psychiatric interviews, neuropsychological tests), the exclusion of causes of dementia other than Alzheimer's disease and vascular dementia, and a differential diagnosis between DAT and VD (ischaemic score, modified ischaemic score including CT and MRI, differentiation of clinical features ascribed to DAT and VD and focal EEG-changes, among others).

Memory loss is a feature of all forms of dementia, including those due to multiple cerebral infarctions. M.M. Cohen, USA, reports that the hippocampal formation, in particular, has been implicated as being critical for recent memory deficits in experimental animals and in humans. Bilateral hippocampal lesions disrupt spatial memory or cognitive mapping in lower mammals and lead to rapid loss of newly acquired information. Ischaemic hippocampal necrosis is a delayed rather than acute event.

Clinically, two broad categories are prominent in chronic cerebrovascular disease. First, patients with severe focal neurological symptoms and often also dementia after a major stroke. Second, patients in whom progressive dementia is the dominant manifestation of cerebrovascular disease.

As it is difficult to distinguish clinically vascular dementia from cases of primary degenerative dementia, N.A. Lassen, Denmark, suggests to add the regional measurement of cerebral blood flow (CBF) and of cerebral metabolic rate of oxygen ($CMRO_2$) to the classical neuroimaging techniques CT and MRI for differential diagnosis.

Here, SPECT provides reliable data indicating that in patients with degenerative dementia either the absence of the cortical parieto-temporal low flow pattern or symmetrical frontal lobe flow can be observed. In vascular dementia, however, asymmetries of cortical CBF occur more frequently.

M.D. O'Brien, United Kingdom, critically discusses the importance of cerebrovascular disease as a cause of dementia as well as the underlying mechanisms. The author urges the need for a more appropriate definition of vascular dementia as the terms multi-infarct dementia and senile dementia might be rather misleading. Besides patients who definitely have a vascular cause of dementia, there exists a group with a mixed type of dementia in which degenerative and vascular pathology co-occur. Such a redefinition will certainly have an influence on the prevalence rate of dementia with vascular pathology.

The author also stresses that cerebrovascular disease causes dementia by a combination of the volume of infarcted tissue, the location of the lesions and, particularly, their bilaterality.

V. Hachinski, Canada, claims that the clinical assessment remains the mainstay and most reliable method of assessing multi-infarct dementia (MID). This involves three overlapping steps, namely determining dementia by clinical history, by physical examination and by mental status scales, determining the type of dementia as well as distinguishing between Alzheimer's disease and MID.

For the latter, the ischemic score remains the single most useful method. Hachinski presents a detailed analysis of the thirteen items and their contribution to the assessment.

The differential diagnosis also comprises the radiological assessment by CT and MRI, as well as the neurophysiological assessment by EEG and short latency somatosensory evoked potentials.

J.P. Blass, USA, outlines the principles of designing clinical trials on vascular dementia. The corresponding clinical criteria were used for a single-centre, double-blind, placebo-controlled trial of pentoxifylline (Trental) in vascular dementia. The patients underwent a treatment with either pentoxifylline or placebo for a period of 36 weeks.

When mean Alzheimer's Disease Assessment Score (ADAS) at the beginning of the trial was compared with the mean score at the end of the trial, there was significant deterioration in the placebo group, while the patients receiving pentoxifylline did not show significant difference from baseline. Pentoxifylline appears to have a positive effect on the course of vascular dementia, significantly slowing the course of deterioration.

The management of chronic cerebrovascular disease is reviewed by H. Lechner, Austria. The underlying strategies focus on the improvement of disturbed cerebral function and the prevention of relapses. Attention should be paid to reducing cerebrovascular risk factors such as smoking habits, arterial hypertension, impaired cardiac function and diabetes. Additionally, a pathological status of haemorheological factors should be corrected by adequate therapeutic measures.

Patients with acute ischaemic stroke or vascular dementia due to multifocal ischaemic lesions represent a heavy burden for the family and society. Although the experimental and clinical investigational tools and diagnostic techniques presently available have reached a most advanced and sophisticated level, the therapeutic measures are still limited and are subject to critical debate.

It was therefore an essential contribution to the XIVth World Congress of Neurology to provide a venue for this state-of-the-art symposium on cerebrovascular disease, documenting facts and shaping the vision of progress.

Contents

Part One

Acute Cerebrovascular Disease

Neuroepidemiology of cerebrovascular disease: An overview*

Bento P.M. Schulte
Institute of Neurology, Catholic University, P.O. Box 9101, 6500 HB Nijmegen, The Netherlands

In developed countries, stroke is the third leading cause of death (after heart disease and cancer), and in many surviving patients, it is the devastating endpoint of cerebrovascular disease (CVD). To date, the best approach to CVD in general, and stroke in particular, is prevention. Rational prevention measures are derived from the data of well-conducted neuroepidemiological studies. During the last three decades, considerable literature describing the epidemiology of CVD has been published. The following is an overview of the neuroepidemiology of CVD for clinical neurologists [1].

Neuroepidemiology is the study of the distribution and determinants of neurological disease in human populations and the factors affecting those characteristics [2]. In designing studies, the most important considerations are representativeness of the population selected for investigation and accuracy of the diagnoses in that population. To correctly analyse the results of epidemiological investigations, one must be familiar with the complete definition of the disease entity being studied. Many but not all studies have defined stroke according to the criteria of the World Health Organisation (WHO) as 'rapidly developing clinical signs of focal (at times global) disturbance of cerebral function, lasting more than 24 h or leading to death with no apparent cause other than that of vascular origin. Transient episodes of cerebral ischaemia were excluded by definition' [3]. The last sentence of the WHO definition is especially important. For proper analysis of the results of epidemiological studies, it is also necessary to know how the subtypes of CVD and stroke were coded. In successive revisions of the WHO International Classification of Diseases (ICD), the same subtype of stroke is sometimes given different three-digit codes [4]. Moreover, in the current 9th revision of the ICD [4], CVD is still listed under the circulatory system, as it may well be in the upcoming 10th revision.

Disease frequency is measured by the following epidemiological indices: mortality, incidence, and prevalence. Descriptive studies using these three indices for CVD provide important information for formulating aetiological hypotheses. These hypotheses are tested using the techniques of analytic epidemiology (case-control or prospective studies). Thus, risk factors associated with CVD are identified. The fact that exclusion of risk factors is beneficial to preventing or reducing

* This paper is written in memory of the late Bruce S. Schoenberg, M.D., Dr P.H., F.A.C.P.

the frequency of CVD can be tested in experimental studies with controlled clinical trials.

Descriptive studies

Mortality

Mortality data have yielded information for large populations worldwide for many years. An official death certificate is required by the government in most nations. Thus, mortality data are collected relatively uniformly, and are available for analysis by age, sex, race, or geographic origin. Despite this advantage, using mortality statistics for establishing the frequency of CVD poses several dilemmas. In such tabulations, those strokes having high case fatality ratios are over-represented. A major problem is the uncertain accuracy of the diagnosis appearing on the death certificate. The death certificate is often rapidly filled out by a poorly informed physician, who may have only been called on to pronounce the patient dead. Diagnoses of stroke subtypes seem correct in only a minority of cases, except for those coded as subarachnoid haemorrhage [5]. Even in the Framingham study, considerable errors for stroke as a whole were made [6]. Another problem is that only one disease per person as the underlying cause of death is allowed on the death certificate. After analysing mortality data from the United States for deaths due to and related to 20 neurologic diseases for 1971 and 1973 through 1978, Chandra et al. [7] concluded that stroke as a single underlying cause of death was under-represented on death certificates.

Fratiglioni et al. [8], using data from 1967 through 1973 for 33 countries, calculated average annual CVD mortality rates, age-adjusted to the 1950 U.S. population. Of these nations, 27 were from Europe and America, only 2 were in Asia (Japan and the Philippines). Rates ranged from 35.8/100,000/year for the Philippines to 196.7/100,000/year for Japan. There was also considerable variation among European and North American countries, with most nations having annual rates close to 100/100,000 (Fig. 1). In the same paper, the rates from 1967 through 1973 were compared to age-adjusted rates from 1951 through 1958, previously calculated for the same 33 countries [9]. Approximately two-thirds of the nations for which data were available showed a marked decline in mortality rates. Of the 22 countries showing such a decline, 11 had a total percentage change of more than 20%. Several other studies reported major decreasing trends in mortality rates from CVD [10–14]. It is suggested that changes in coding conventions and inaccuracies on the death certificate explain the downward trend in mortality rates but this has not been verified. Garland et al. [15] described the trends in mortality rates from CVD in Baltimore, Maryland, during 1950–1970 with reference to all information found in the medical records. Overall accuracy of death certificate diagnoses did not change markedly during the study period. These investigators concluded that the decline of death rates could not be solely attributed to errors in death certificate diagnoses (Fig. 2).

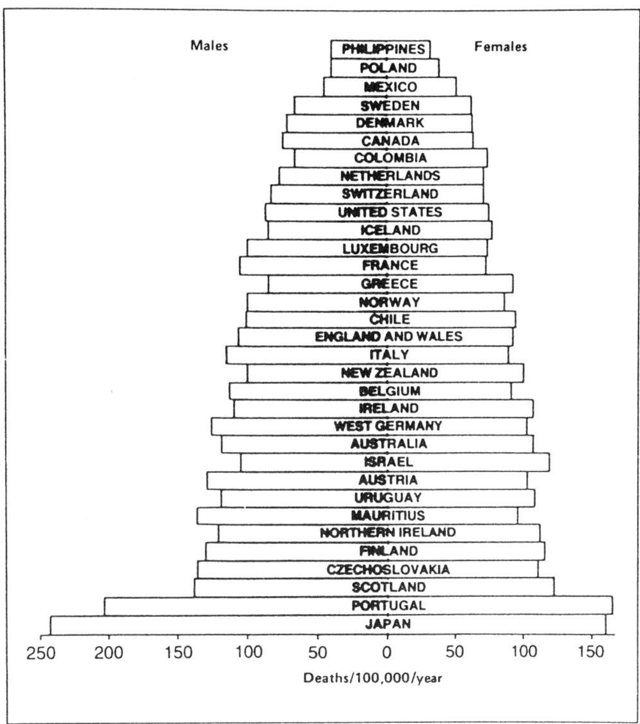

Fig. 1. Average annual age-adjusted (to 1950 United States population) mortality rates (per 100,000), by sex, for cerebrovascular disease, 1967–1973. Reproduced from Fratiglioni et al. [8], by courtesy of the Publishers.

Yatsu et al. [16] found lower mortality rates in three community hospital-based stroke programs in the United States during 1979–1980 than in the National Survey of Stroke during 1975–1976 [17]. It appeared that stroke severity was less in the former than in the latter study. This finding agreed with the hypothesis that the national decline in stroke mortality may be partly due to a decline in stroke severity rather than simply to a decline in incidence. Strong evidence exists, however, that the decline in stroke mortality should be attributed to better control of severe and moderate, and even mild, hypertension [18–20]. The phenomenon of a downward trend in stroke mortality even before hypertension was pharmacologically treated may be explained in the United States by changes in lifestyle [21] and by lower salt intake since the early decades of this century [22].

For all types of CVD, some general characteristics are applicable. Age-specific mortality rates rise steeply with increasing age [5,23]. Mortality rates analysed by sex revealed only a slight male excess for stroke in contrast to the strong male preponderance in mortality from ischaemic heart disease [8]. Before age 55, the male: female ratio for all stroke subtypes is high, at least in Sweden [24]. Although it has long been recognised that blacks in the United States have higher stroke death rates than whites of the same age and sex living in the same geographic

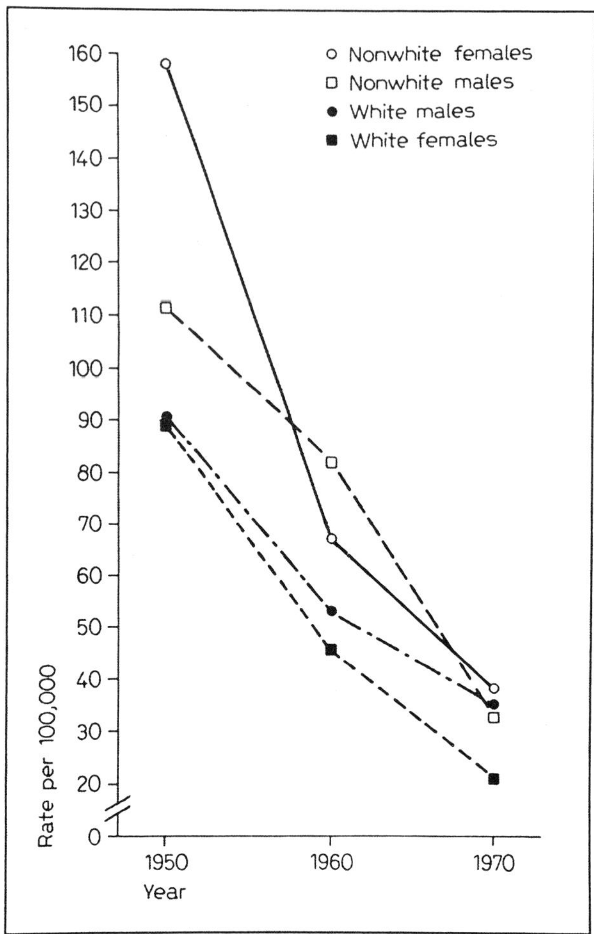

Fig. 2. Annual age-adjusted (to 1960 United States population) mortality rates per 100,000 population for cerebral hemorrhage (ICDA 8th revision, code 431), Baltimore, Maryland, 1950, 1960 and 1970. Reproduced from Garland et al. [15] by courtesy of the Publishers.

region, the reason for this discrepancy is still unknown [7,25]. There are geographic differences in mortality from stroke in the United States, Japan, the People's Republic of China, and France. In the United States, stroke mortality maps for three 7-year periods between 1962 and 1982 for U.S. whites aged 35–74 years showed an east-west gradient of high-to-low stroke mortality rates [26]. In Japan, age-adjusted mortality rates for CVD are higher in northeastern areas than in the southwestern part of the country [27]. In the People's Republic of China, age adjusted mortality rates from urban areas are highest in the northeast and lowest in the southwest [28]. The geographic pattern of stroke mortality in France did not change during 1962–1982; the highest rates were always found in the southwestern part of the country and in Bretagne for both sexes [29].

Incidence and prevalence

As has been mentioned, stroke mortality data contain many potential biases. The best measure of stroke risk is incidence. Because of differences in experimental design worldwide, data from incidence studies must be cautiously compared. Hospital-based investigations cannot precisely identify a population at risk, and it is impossible to calculate rates [30,31]. Furthermore, hospital-based studies may not be representative of all cases of CVD in the community. Since patients with severe strokes are more likely to be admitted to hospital, the distribution of stroke subtypes in the population may be incorrectly reflected [32]. Incidence rates derived from hospital data may underestimate the frequency of first completed stroke by 25–30% [33]. In a well-designed population-based incidence study such bias is excluded. But even in population-based investigations, there are differences that must be considered before making any comparisons. While some studies include all forms of CVD, others include only completed strokes; some count all episodes of stroke, and others exclude all but the first-ever stroke. Many community-based stroke incidence studies have been carried out in Europe, North America, Asia, Africa, and Australia. Recently, in a survey of CVD, Kurtzke [34] compared incidence rates of first completed stroke based on community studies from North America, western Europe, and Australia. After age-adjusting the incidence rates to the 1960 U.S. population, the resulting figures ranged from 100–250 new cases/100,000/year. Because many stroke incidence studies differ in design, comparisons between them may be invalid. In order to improve this situation, Malmgren et al. [35] proposed criteria for the 'ideal' stroke study. These criteria include the following: standard diagnostic criteria (according to the WHO); complete case ascertainment; prospective study design; definition of incident cases of those patients with their first-ever stroke; classification of a pathological type of stroke; rates given for all pathological types of stroke combined; well-defined denominator; representative and large population; rates calculated for similar time periods; cases collected for whole years; standard presentation of rates by age, sex, and race. Fifty-six published stroke incidence studies failed to meet these criteria. Nine comparable incidence studies remained: 5 in Europe, 1 each in the United States, New-Zealand, Japan, and Libya [36–44]. Only three time-trend studies came close to the ideal [38,43–45].

The percentages of the specific stroke subtypes in stroke incidence studies must be carefully evaluated, especially those performed before the introduction of computed tomography (CT). Wherever population studies of completed stroke have been carried out, cerebral infarction accounts for the majority of the incident cases. In a community-based study of a Caucasian population, Kurtzke [46] estimated that 8% of strokes are due to subarachnoid haemorrhage; 12% to intracranial haemorrhage; 69% to thromboembolic infarction; and 11% to ill-defined strokes. In the Harvard Cooperative Stroke Registry, 6% of all strokes are due to subarachnoid haemorrhage; 10% to intracranial haemorrhage; and 82% to thromboembolic infarction [47]. In population-based studies from Japan [42] and the People's Republic of China [28], the proportion of intracerebral haemorrhage is considerably higher when compared with Caucasian populations. Although strokes occur during every stage of life [48], incidence rates for stroke increase exponentially with age, both in Caucasian [5] and Oriental populations [28]. Most stroke incidence studies suggest a slight male excess [49]. In a recent study, however, Terent [50] reported an increase in stroke incidence among Swedish women during 1975–1978 and 1983–1986. The increased risk among men, as reported in most studies is far below the male excess for myocardial infarction [51].

Blacks have higher stroke incidence rates than whites, at least in the United States. In several studies, black women had higher incidence rates than white women in each group; and black men had higher incidence rates than white men up to age 75 [25].

With regard to geographic variation, Japan [52] and the northeastern region of the People's Republic of China [28] reported the highest incidence rates for stroke. Research on Japanese migrants indicated the highest stroke prevalence in Japanese men in Japan, intermediate rates for Japanese in Hawaii, and lowest for Japanese living in California [53]. It is suggested that environmental factors are related to geographic variations, and that dietary animal protein and fat exert an inhibitory effect on stroke incidence [54]. The data on geographic variation must be interpreted cautiously. After analysis of 65 published stroke incidence studies, Malmgren et al. [35] concluded that geographic differences in stroke incidence are not very great. Alter et al. [55] calculated age- and sex-standardised incidence ratios of stroke in 13 countries from 6 continents based on recent reports. These authors also concluded that the worldwide variation in the age- and sex-adjusted stroke rates is relatively small (Fig. 3).

Since the late 1950s, incidence rates for stroke have been declining, at least in Japan [45,56] and in the United States [38,57,58]. In Hisayama, Japan, the annual age-adjusted rate per 1000 person-years for cerebral haemorrhage decreased by 29% between 1961–1966 and 1972–1976. The rate for cerebral infarction fell significantly by 34% over the same time period, especially in females [45]. A time-trend study in Framingham, Massachusetts, where uniform criteria and case ascertainment have been maintained for more than three decades, showed a decline in stroke incidence but only in women [58]. Conclusive evidence that stroke incidence is diminishing came from Rochester, Minnesota, U.S.A. Comparison of quinquennia from 1945 through 1979 showed a 54% decrease of all first-ever strokes [38]. Homer et al. [59] extended the observations back through 1935 in the same population. The trend in the incidence of stroke for women did not change from 1935 to 1954, after which there was a gradual decline. For men, there was little change until 1969, after which there was a sharp decline (Fig. 4). With the exception of improved detection and treatment of hypertension, suggestions offered to explain the decrease in stroke incidence remain speculative [60]. On the basis of data from the Rochester, Minnesota population, Garraway and Whisnant [61] concluded that improvements in detecting and controlling hypertension during 1950–1979 accounted for the declining incidence of stroke in that population (Fig. 5).

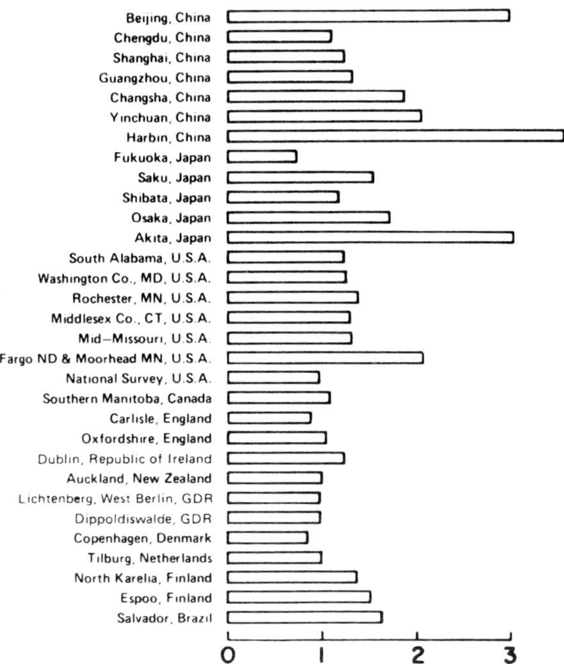

Fig. 3. Age-specific standardised incidence ratios, based on the 1976 United States population, for initial stroke in selected communities. Reproduced from Alter et al. [55] by courtesy of the Publishers.

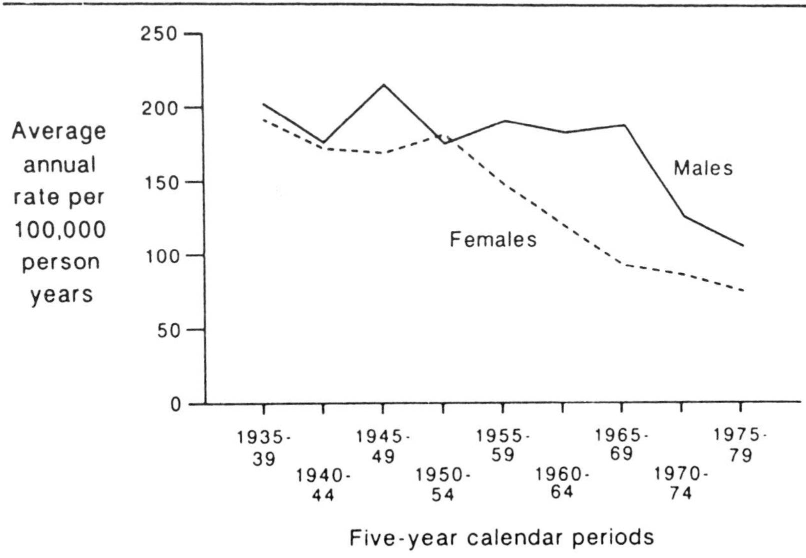

Fig. 4. Sex-specific temporal trends in the age-adjusted (to 1950 United States white population) incidence rates of completed stroke in Rochester, Minnesota, 1935–1979. Reproduced from Homer et al. [59] by courtesy of the Publishers.

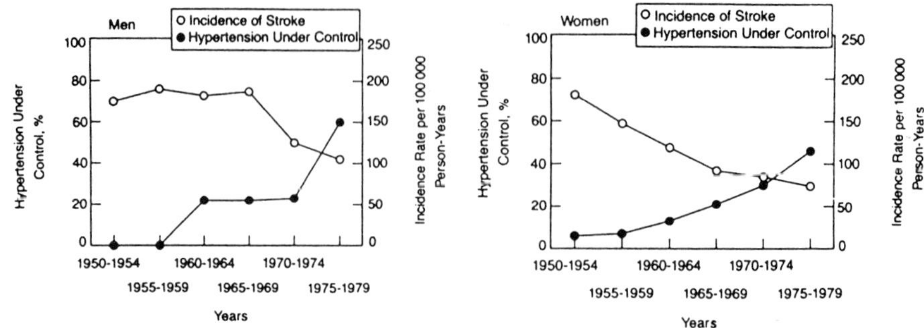

Fig. 5. Average annual age-adjusted (to 1950 United States white population) incidence rates for stroke in Rochester, Minnesota, and percentage of persons with hypertension under control (diastolic blood pressure < 95 mmHg) in various periods in men and women. Reproduced from Garraway and Whisnant [61] by courtesy of the Publishers.

Reliable data on prevalence of CVD and stroke are scarce. Much quoted data are those of the National Survey of Stroke, organised in the 1970s in the United States. The National Survey average 1976 age-specific prevalence rates were 743/100,000 for all ages; for those under 45 years, 66/100,000; from 45 through 65 years, 998/100,000; and for those over age 65, 5,063/100,000 [62]. Using a WHO protocol, prevalence studies have been carried out in the United States, Ecuador, Mexico, Nigeria, the People's Republic of China, and Peru [63]. In general, the prevalence ratio for CVD throughout the world is about 500–700/100,000 [46,64]. High prevalence ratios were found among men in Finland [65] and the Parsi in Bombay, India [66].

Despite declining rates, stroke is a major cause of mortality and morbidity. There is little expectation that better management of stroke will substantially diminish the outcome of CVD. Therefore, it is essential to prevent stroke by identifying the stroke-prone individual. The study of factors that increase the risk of stroke is the domain of analytic neuroepidemiology.

Analytic studies

From the results of several previous case-control studies and few prospective investigations, a profile of the stroke-prone individual is emerging. Age is the most powerful risk factor for stroke; above age 55, the risk of having a stroke doubles with each decade. Another untreatable risk factor is sex; men, especially under age 65, have a 30% higher incidence than women.

Among treatable risk factors, hypertension is the most important and highly prevalent risk factor (Table 1). Moreover, the attributable risk is highest for hypertension as well. The risk of stroke rises with increasing blood pressure, not only among hypertensives but for all ranges of blood pressure. Isolated systolic hypertension is also a risk factor [10,67–71]. The presence of various types of heart

Table 1. Common currently recognized risk factors for cerebrovascular disease

Hypertension
Heart disease
Transient ischaemic attacks
Diabetes mellitus
Obesity (not independent)
Exogenous estrogens
Cigarette smoking
Alcohol consumption
Prior stroke

disease increases the risk of stroke. Cardiac impairments which contribute independently to stroke include left ventricular hypertrophy on ECG, cardiac enlargement on X-ray, coronary heart disease, myocardial infarction, congestive heart failure, and atrial fibrillation. Other cardiac disorders, such as chronic rheumatic valvular disease, infective and marantic endocarditis, prolapsed mitral valve, and cardiac myxoma, are also associated with an increased risk of embolic stroke [67]. Diabetes mellitus is an important risk factor for stroke in general, and cerebral infarction in particular. In the Framingham study, it was a most important predictive factor [67]. Transient ischaemic attacks (TIAs) are an important risk factor for completed ischaemic stroke. Only 10% of strokes, however, are preceded by TIAs. The risk of stroke appears to be increased tenfold in those who have experienced TIAs. More than 35% can expect a stroke within 4 years [44,72]. Analysis of the published data of 34 studies of the long-term prognosis after TIAs indicated that, from approximately one year after TIA onset, the hazard rate is approximately constant and the level of excess annual mortality relative to the general population's experience is approximately 85% [73].

A relationship between elevated serum lipids and lipoproteins is not well established for CVD. Prospective studies in the United States could not document an association between serum triglycerides and completed ischaemic stroke [74]. The relationship between serum cholesterol levels and stroke is also equivocal. In the Framingham study, there was a negative relationship between low-density lipoproteins (LDL)-cholesterol blood levels and the risk of stroke, especially in women [67]. It has been shown recently that stroke itself lowers serum lipid levels [75]. In other studies, serum cholesterol level was either confirmed [76] or not confirmed [77] as a risk factor for stroke.

Obesity does not seem to be an independent risk factor for stroke [10]. However, it is a major risk factor for elevated blood pressure and diabetes. If there is an association between obesity and stroke, it may be the result of concurrent hypertension and elevated blood glucose levels [74].

The use of exogenous estrogens, either in women taking oral contraceptives [78] or in men with prostate cancer treated with high-dose estrogen [79] is associated with an increased risk of stroke. Regarding contraceptives, the relative risk is great but the absolute risk is small. The risk is enhanced by age, coexisting hypertension, migraine, diabetes, hyperlipidaemia, and cigarette smoking. In recent years the role of oral contraceptives as a risk factor for stroke has been questioned. There may be a tendency for physicians to over-diagnose a neurologic illness as a 'stroke' when confronted with a patient currently taking oral contraceptives [67]. After analysing the literature, Kurtzke [68] concluded that oral contraceptives play no significant role in stroke genesis, at least of thrombotic strokes.

Until recently, an association between cigarette smoking and an increased risk of stroke had been demonstrated only for subarachnoid haemorrhage [80,81]. For other types of stroke, the data were inconsistent [10,68]. From the Framingham data, it was concluded that, although the impact of cigarette smoking was modest, marginally significant, and confined to men below age 65, the effect where it existed was an independent one, not accounted for by the associated risk factors [67]. However, recent studies have changed this. The results of a retrospective case-control study indicated that a cumulative lifetime exposure to active cigarette smoking was directly associated with CVD [82]. Cigarette smoking was correlated with an increased incidence of both thromboembolic and haemorrhagic strokes in a study of Hawaiian men of Japanese ancestry, with no diminution with advancing age. The cessation of cigarette smoking after many years of smoking was associated with a significantly lower risk of stroke than persistent smoking in this male population [83,84]. A strong causal relationship between cigarette smoking and stroke among young and middle-aged women was found in a prospective cohort study of women 30–55 years of age and free from coronary heart disease, stroke, and cancer [85]. Recent data from the Framingham study indicated that cigarette smoking significantly and independently contributed to the risk of stroke in general and infarction in particular, after accounting for age and hypertension [86].

Results regarding alcohol consumption have been equivocal. The Framingham data suggested a statistically insignificant association between alcohol intake and stroke in men [67,68]. In the Honolulu Heart Study, a correlation was found between haemorrhagic stroke and alcohol consumption, which was largely associated with hypertension and smoking [87]. In other investigations, there was no significant effect of alcohol intake on stroke occurrence [76,88]. In a recent review of the literature, it was concluded that regular alcohol ingestion is associated with hypertension, fatal and nonfatal intracranial haemorrhage, cerebral infarction, and increased risk of death from stroke [89]. The influence of alcohol use on the risk of stroke depends on the amount of alcohol consumed [84]. Among men, the relative risk of stroke was lower in light drinkers than in nondrinkers, but was four times higher in heavy drinkers than in nondrinkers [90]. These data from a case-control study need to be confirmed in a prospective study [84]. Results from a prospective study suggest that among middle-aged women, moderate alcohol consumption decreases the risk of ischaemic stroke but may increase the risk of subarachnoid haemorrhage [91].

Prior stroke must be considered a major risk factor [92]. Other risk factors such as sickle cell anaemia, collagen vascular disease, polycythaemia, and elevated haemoglobin level have a low prevalence. Many risk factors are poorly documented, e.g., personality, lifestyle, type of work, socioeconomic status, heredity, migraine headaches, diet, coffee-drinking, soft water, low altitude, low environmental temperature, seasonal variation [10,67,68]. Despite this array of risk factors, we still cannot adequately explain the large proportion of strokes that occur. Many currently recognised risk factors are poorly understood and unknown risk factors remain to be discovered.

Experimental studies

By using the experimental epidemiological techniques of controlled clinical trials, it is possible to make rational decisions about the usefulness and safety of new drugs and procedures. A clinical trial is a prospective study in human subjects comparing the effect and value of intervention(s) with a control condition [93]. Despite multiple difficulties in designing and implementing these investigations, there are several reports describing successful large-scale application of these techniques to clinically relevant questions related to CVD. This is illustrated by the following medical and surgical trials.

The results of several important clinical trials for treating hypertension have clearly demonstrated the efficacy of therapy in reducing the incidence of stroke, especially cerebral haemorrhage [10]. Twelve randomised clinical trials of antihypertensive therapy were recently reviewed by Furberg et al. [93]. In all trials, there was a demonstrable reduction in stroke incidence in the treated subjects. Among these trials, the study of the multicentred Hypertension Detection and Follow-up Program Cooperative Group [94] deserves special mention. In this community-based, randomised controlled clinical trial, systematic stepped care therapy (i.e., patients actively treated) was compared with referred care therapy (i.e., patients referred back to their own physician) in hypertensives. In 1982, the stepped care 5-year stroke incidence was significantly lower than that found among the referred care patients, and the CVD mortality decreased in the stepped care population to a level approaching that of the general United States population. Although the design of several antihypertensive therapy trials has been criticised [69], they are still examples of the usefulness of experimental epidemiology.

In the last decade, there have been many clinical trials of antiplatelet agents for secondary prevention of ischaemic cerebral or myocardial events. Aspirin is now recognised as effective in the secondary prevention of strokes and heart attacks. A noteworthy study in the United Kingdom reported a significant 18% reduction of nonfatal myocardial infarction, nonfatal major stroke, vascular death, or nonvascular death in patients receiving aspirin. While the reduction was partly due to an unexpected decrease in nonvascular death and vascular endpoints were not significantly lowered, this trial is important because there was no obvious difference between responses to the 300 mg and 1200 mg daily aspirin doses, except that the lower dose was considerably less gastrotoxic [95]. In a recent review, data were pooled for 25 randomised clinical trials of antiplatelet treatment for patients with a history of TIAs, occlusive stroke, unstable angina, or myocardial infarction [96]. Drug treatment significantly reduced vascular mortality by 15% and nonfatal vascular events (stroke and myocardial infarction) by 30%. There was no significant difference between the effects of the different types of antiplatelet treatment tested. Aspirin in a daily dose of 300 mg was as effective as when taken in larger amounts.

Regarding the possible preventive effect of surgical therapy, the following clinical trials must be mentioned. Since 1967, the application of extracranial-intracranial arterial bypass for symptomatic but conventionally inoperable extracranial vascular disease was advocated on the basis of uncontrolled studies or anecdotal evidence only. In a large international prospective randomised clinical trial, the Extracranial-Intracranial (EC/IC) Bypass Study Group [97] showed no benefit related to stroke prevention or death following anastomosis of the superficial temporal artery to the middle cerebral artery in patients with atherosclerotic arterial disease in the carotid and middle cerebral arteries. Although the conclusions were criticised because 50–70% of eligible patients were not included in the study [98], this trial underlines the importance of experimental epidemiology.

Since 1954, carotid endarterectomy has been performed on an ever-larger scale as a surgical procedure for preventing of stroke and death in patients with TIAs or even in those with asymptomatic carotid bruits. In the mid-1980s, the possible benefits of this technique have been increasingly criticised [99]. In response to this criticism, several large multicentre controlled clinical trials are now underway in Europe and North America [100]. The results of these trials will undoubtedly influence the attitude of the medical community with regard to this surgical procedure.

Acknowledgements

The author is indebted to Mrs Devera G. Schoenberg, B.S., M.S., for critically reading and editing the manuscript, and to Mrs Marlies Peters-van den Ing for secretarial assistance.

References

1. Schoenberg BS and Schulte BPM (1988) Cerebrovascular disease: epidemiology and geopathology. In: Vinken PJ, Bruyn GW and Klawans HL (eds.) Handbook of clinical neurology, vol. 53, revised series vol. 9, Toole JF (co-ed.). Elsevier Science Publishers, Amsterdam, pp. 1–26.
2. Schoenberg BS (1982) The scope of neuroepidemiology: From stone-age to Stockholm. Neuroepidemiology 1: 1–16.
3. Hatano S (1976) Experience from a multicentre stroke register: A preliminary report. Bull. WHO 54: 541–553.
4. WHO (1948 6th rev., 1957 7th rev., 1967 8th rev., 1977 9th rev.) International statistical classification of diseases, injuries and causes of death. WHO, Geneva.

5. Kurtzke JF (1969) Epidemiology of cerebrovascular disease. Springer, Berlin.
6. Corwin LI, Wolf PA, Kannel WB and McNamara PM (1982) Accuracy of death certification of stroke: The Framingham Study. Stroke 13: 818–821.
7. Chandra V, Bharucha NE and Schoenberg BS (1984) Mortality data for the US for deaths due to and related to twenty neurological diseases. Neuroepidemiology 3: 149–168.
8. Fratiglioni L, Massey EW, Schoenberg DG and Schoenberg BS (1983) Mortality from cerebrovascular disease: International comparisons and temporal trends. Neuroepidemiology 2: 101–16.
9. Goldberg ID and Kurland LT (1962) Mortality in 33 countries from diseases of the nervous system. World Neurol. 3: 444–465.
10. Kuller LH (1978) Epidemiology of stroke. In: Schoenberg BS (ed.) Neurological epidemiology: principles and clinical applications. Raven Press, New York, pp. 281–311.
11. Ostfeld AM (1980) A review of stroke epidemiology. Epidemiol. Rev. 2: 136–152.
12. Prineas RJ (1971) Cerebrovascular disease occurrence in Australia. Med. J. Austr. 2: 509–515.
13. Soltero I, Liu K, Cooper R, Stamler J and Garside D (1978) Trends in mortality from cerebrovascular diseases in the United States, 1960–1975. Stroke 9: 549–555.
14. Wylic CM (1961) Cerebrovascular accident deaths in the United States and in England and Wales. J. Chronic Dis. 15: 85–90.
15. Garland FC, Lilienfeld AM and Garland CF (1989) Declining trends in mortality from cerebrovascular disease at ages 10–65 years: A test of validity. Neuroepidemiology 8: 1–23.
16. Yatsu FM, Becker C, McLeroy KR, Coull B, Feibel J, Howard G, Toole JF and Walker MD (1986) Community hospital-based stroke programs: North Carolina, Oregon, and New York. I. Goals, objectives and data collection procedures. Stroke 17: 276–284.
17. Walker AE, Robins M and Weinfeld FD (1981) Clinical findings. In: Weinfeld FD (ed.) The National Survey of Stroke. Stroke 12 (suppl. 1): I-13–44.
18. Veterans Administration Cooperative Study Group on Antihypertensive Agents (1967) Effects of treatment on morbidity in hypertension: Results in patients with diastolic blood pressures averaging 115 through 129 mmHg. J.A.M.A. 202: 1028–1034.
19. Veterans Administration Cooperative Study Group on Antihypertensive Agents (1970) Effects of treatment on morbidity in hypertension: II. Results in patients with diastolic blood pressure averaging 90 through 114 mmHg. J.A.M.A. 213: 1143–1152.
20. The Australian Therapeutic Trial in Mild Hypertension (1980) Report by the Management Committee. Lancet I: 1261–1267.
21. Walker WJ (1983) Changing US life style and declining vascular mortality – a retrospective. N. Engl. J. Med. 308: 649-651.
22. Joossens JV, Kesteloot H and Amery A (1979) Salt intake and mortality from stroke. N. Engl. J. Med. 300: 1396.
23. Wang CC, Cheng XM, Li SZ, Bolis CL and Schoenberg BS (1983) Epidemiology of cerebrovascular disease in an urban community of Beijing, People's Republic of China. Neuroepidemiology 2: 121–134.
24. Mettinger KL, Söderström CE and Allander E (1984) Epidemiology of acute cerebrovascular disease before the age of 55 in the Stockholm County 1973–1977: I. Incidence and mortality rates. Stroke 15: 795–801.
25. Gillum RF (1988) Stroke in blacks. Stroke 19: 1–9.
26. Wing S, Casper M, Davis WB, Pellom A, Riggan W and Tyroler HA (1988) Stroke mortality maps United States whites aged 35–74 years, 1962–1982. Stroke 19: 1507–1513.
27. Kojima S (1976) Practical aspects of hypertension and stroke control in a rural population. In: Hatano S, Shigematsu I and Strasser T (eds.) Hypertension and stroke control in the community. WHO, Geneva, pp. 149–174.
28. Li SC, Schoenberg BS, Wang CC, Cheng XM, Bolis CL and Wang KJ (1985) Cerebrovascular disease in the People's Republic of China: Epidemiological and clinical features. Neurology 35: 1708–1713.
29. Alpérovitch A, Mas JL, Doyon B and Myquel P (1986) Mortality from stroke in France 1968–1982. Neuroepidemiology 5: 80–87.

30. Bogousslavsky J, Melle G van and Regli F (1988) The Lausanne Stroke Registry: Analysis of 1,000 consecutive patients with first stroke. Stroke 19: 1083–1092.
31. Rosman KD (1986) The epidemiology of stroke in an urban black population. Stroke 17: 667–669.
32. Bamford J, Sandercock P, Warlow C and Gray M (1986) Who are patients with acute stroke admitted to hospital? Br. Med. J. 292: 1369–1372.
33. Schoenberg B, Schoenberg D and Whisnant J (1983) Hospitalization for stroke. A population study in Rochester, Minnesota. Am. J. Epidemiol. 118: 444.
34. Kurtzke JF (1985) Epidemiology of cerebrovascular disease. In: McDowell FH and Caplan LR (eds.) Cerebrovascular survey report for the National Institute of Neurological and Communicative Disorders and Stroke. NINCDS, Bethesda, pp. 1–34.
35. Malmgren R, Bamford J, Warlow C and Sandercock P (1987) Geographical and secular trends in stroke incidence. Lancet II: 1196–1200.
36. Ashok PP, Radhakrishnan K, Sridharan R and El-Mangoush MA (1986) Incidence and pattern of cerebrovascular diseases in Benghazi, Libya. J. Neurol. Neurosurg. Psychiatry 49: 519–523.
37. Bonita R (1986) Cigarette smoking, hypertension and the risk of subarachnoid haemorrhage: A population-based case-control study. Stroke 17: 831–835.
38. Garraway WM, Whisnant JP and Drury I (1983a) The continuing decline in the incidence of stroke. Mayo Clin. Proc. 58: 520–523.
39. Herman B, Leyten ACM, Luijk JH van, Frenken CWGM, Op de Coul AAW and Schulte BPM (1982) Epidemiology of stroke in Tilburg, The Netherlands: The population-based stroke incidence register. 2. Incidence, initial clinical picture and medical care, and three-week case fatality. Stroke 13: 629–634.
40. Kotila M (1984) Declining incidence and mortality of stroke? Stroke 15: 255–259.
41. Oxfordshire Community Stroke Project (1983) Incidence of stroke in Oxfordshire: First year's experience of a community stroke register. Br. Med. J. 287: 713–717.
42. Tanaka H (1982) Age-specific incidence of stroke subtype in Shibata, Japan: 1976–1978. Stroke 13: 110.
43. Terent A (1979) A prospective epidemiological survey of cerebrovascular disease in a Swedish community. Ups. J. Med. Sci. 84: 235–246.
44. Terent A (1986) Hjärnblödning och hjarninfarkt (stroke): Diagnostik och behandling. Medicinska Forskningsradet: 15–26.
45. Ueda K, Omae T, Hirota Y, Takeshita M, Katsuki S, Tanaka K and Enjoji M (1981) Decreasing trend in incidence and mortality from stroke in Hisayama residents, Japan. Stroke 12: 154–160.
46. Kurtzke JF (1980) Epidemiology of cerebrovascular disease. In: Siekert RG (ed.) Cerebrovascular survey report for joint council subcommittee on cerebrovascular disease, NINCDS and National Heart and Lung Institute. Whiting Press, Rochester, pp. 135–176.
47. Mohr JP, Caplan LR, Melski JW, Goldstein RJ, Duncan GW, Kistler JP, Pessin MS and Bleich HL (1978) The Harvard Cooperative Stroke Registry: A prospective registry. Neurology 28: 754–762.
48. Salam-Adams M and Adams RD (1988) Cerebrovascular disease by age group. In: Vinken PJ, Bruyn GW and Klawans HL (eds.) Handbook of clinical neurology, vol. 53, revised series vol. 9, Toole JF (co-ed.). Elsevier Science Publishers, Amsterdam, pp. 27–46.
49. Haberman S, Capildeo R and Rose FC (1981) Sex differences in the incidence of cerebrovascular disease. J. Epidemiol. Community Health 35: 45–50.
50. Terent A (1988) Increasing incidence of stroke among Swedish women. Stroke 19: 598–603.
51. Garraway WM, Elveback LR, Connolly DC and Whisnant JP (1983b) The dichotomy of myocardial and cerebral infarction. Lancet II: 1332–1335.
52. Tanaka H, Ueda Y, Date C, Baba T, Yamashita H, Hayashi M, Shoji H, Owada K, Baba KI, Shibuya M, Kon T and Detels R (1981) Incidence of stroke in Shibata, Japan: 1976–1978. Stroke 12: 460–466.
53. Kagan A, Popper J, Rhoads GG, Takeya Y, Kato H, Goode GB and Marmot M (1976) Epidemiological studies of coronary heart disease and stroke in Japanese men living in Japan, Hawaii, and California: Prevalence of stroke. In: Scheinberg P (ed.) Cerebrovascular diseases. Raven Press, New York, pp. 267–277.

54. Takeya Y, Popper JS, Shimizu Y, Kato H, Rhoads GG and Kagan A (1984) Epidemiological studies of coronary heart disease and stroke in Japanese men living in Japan, Hawaii, and California: Incidence of stroke in Japan and Hawaii. Stroke 15: 15–23.
55. Alter M, Zhang ZX, Sobel E, Fisher M, Davanipour Z and Friday G (1986) Standardised incidence ratios of stroke: A worldwide review. Neuroepidemiology 5: 148–158.
56. Komachi Y, Tanaka H, Shimamoto T, Handa K, Iida M, Isomura K, Kojima S, Matsuzaki T, Ozawa H, Takahashi H and Tsunetoshi Y (1984) A collaborative study of stroke incidence in Japan: 1975–1979. Stroke 15: 28–36.
57. Garraway WM, Whisnant JP, Furlan AJ, Phillips LH, Kurland LT and O'Fallon WM (1979) The declining incidence of stroke. N. Engl. J. Med. 300: 449–452.
58. Wolf PA, Dawber TR, Thomas HE, Colton T, Nickerson R and Pool J (1978a) The declining incidence of stroke: The Framingham Study. Stroke 9: 97.
59. Homer D, Whisnant JP and Schoenberg BS (1987) Trends in the incidence rates of stroke in Rochester, Minnesota, since 1935. Ann. Neurol. 22: 245–251.
60. Whisnant JP (1984) The decline of stroke. Stroke 15: 160–168.
61. Garraway WM and Whisnant JP (1987) The changing pattern of hypertension and the declining incidence of stroke. J.A.M.A. 258: 214–217.
62. Baum HM and Robins M (1981) Survival and prevalence. In: Weinfeld FD (ed.) The National Survey of Stroke. Stroke (suppl. 1) 12: I-59–68.
63. Schoenberg BS (1983) Neuroepidemiologic generalizations: High tax on importing data, low tax on importing principles. Neuroepidemiology 2: 117–120.
64. Kurtzke JF (1982) The current neurologic burden of illness and injury in the United States. Neurology 32: 1207–1214.
65. Aho K, Reunanen A, Aromaa A, Knekt P and Maatela J (1986) Prevalence of stroke in Finland. Stroke 17: 681–686.
66. Bharucha NE, Bharucha EP, Bharucha AE, Bhise AV and Schoenberg BS (1988) Prevalence of stroke in the Parsi community of Bombay. Stroke 19: 60–62.
67. Kannel WB and Wolf PA (1983) Epidemiology of cerebrovascular disease. In: Ross Russel RW (ed.) Vascular disease of the central nervous system. Churchill Livingstone, Edinburgh, pp. 1–24.
68. Kurtzke JF (1983) Epidemiology and risk factors in thrombotic brain infarction. In: Harrison MJG and Dyken ML (eds.) Cerebral vascular disease. Butterworths, London, pp. 27–45.
69. Mitchell JRA (1983) Hypertension and stroke. In: Harrison MJG and Dyken ML (eds.) Cerebral vascular disease. Butterworths, London, pp. 46–66.
70. Wolf PA, Kannel WB and Dawber TR (1978b) Prospective investigations: The Framingham Study and the epidemiology of stroke. In: Schoenberg BS (ed.) Neurological epidemiology: Principles and clinical applications. Raven Press, New York, pp. 107–120.
71. Wolf PA, Dawber TR and Kannel WB (1978c) Heart disease as a precursor of stroke. In: Schoenberg BS (ed.) Neurological epidemiology: Principles and clinical applications. Raven Press, New York, pp. 567–577.
72. Loeb C and Gandolfo C (1988) Transient ischaemic neurological deficits. In: Vinken PJ, Bruyn GW and Klawans HL (eds.) Handbook of clinical neurology, vol. 53, revised series vol. 9, Toole JF (co-ed.). Elsevier Science Publishers, Amsterdam, pp. 257–290.
73. Haberman S (1984) Long-term prognosis after transient ischaemic attacks. Neuroepidemiology 3: 108–128.
74. Wolf PA, Kannel WB and Verter J (1983) Current status of risk factors for stroke. Neurol. Clin. 1: 317–343.
75. Mendez I, Hachinski V and Wolfe B (1987) Serum lipids after stroke. Neurology 37: 507–511.
76. Boysen G, Nyboe J, Appleyard M, Soelberg Sørensen P, Boas J, Somnier F, Jensen G and Schnohr P (1988) Stroke incidence and risk factors for stroke in Copenhagen, Denmark. Stroke 19: 1345–1353.
77. Welin L, Svärdsudd K, Wilhelmsen L, Larsson B and Tibblin G (1987) Analysis of risk factors for stroke in a cohort of men born in 1913. N. Engl. J. Med. 317: 521–526.
78. Collaborative Group for the Study of Stroke in Young Women (1973) Oral contraception and increased risk of cerebral ischemia or thrombosis. N. Engl. J. Med. 288: 871–878.

79. Veterans Administration Cooperative Urological Research Group (1967) Treatment and survival of patients with cancer of the prostate. Surg. Gynecol. Obstet. 124: 1011–1017.
80. Bonita R, Beaglehole R and North JDK (1984) Event, incidence and case fatality rates of cerebrovascular disease in Auckland, New Zealand. Am. J. Epidemiol. 120: 236–243.
81. Sacco RL, Wolf PA, Bharucha NE, Meeks SL, Kannel WB, Charette LJ, McNamara PM, Palmer EP and D'Agostino R (1984) Subarachnoid and intracerebral hemorrhage: natural history, prognosis and precursive factors in the Framingham Study. Neurology 34: 847–854.
82. Molgaard CA, Bartok A, Peddecord KM and Rothrock J (1986) The association between cerebrovascular disease and smoking: A case-control study. Neuroepidemiology 5: 88–94.
83. Abbott RD, Yin Y, Reed DM and Yano K (1986) Risk of stroke in male cigarette smokers. N. Engl. J. Med. 315: 717–720.
84. Wolf PA (1986) Cigarettes, alcohol and stroke. N. Engl. J. Med. 315: 1087–1089.
85. Colditz GA, Bonita R, Stampfer MJ, Willett WC, Rosner B, Speizer FE and Hennekens CH (1988) Cigarette smoking and risk of stroke in middle-aged women. N. Engl. J. Med. 318: 937–941.
86. Wolf PA, D'Agostino RB, Kannel WB, Bonita R and Belanger AJ (1988) Cigarette smoking as a risk factor for stroke: the Framingham Study. J.A.M.A. 259: 1025–1029.
87. Blackwelder WC, Yano K, Rhoads GG, Kagan A, Gordon T and Palesch Y (1980) Alcohol and mortality: The Honolulu Heart Study. Am. J. Med. 68: 164–169.
88. Herman B, Schmitz PIM, Leyten ACM, Luijk JH van, Frenken CWGM, Op de Coul AAW and Schulte BPM (1983) Multivariate logistic analysis of risk factors for stroke in Tilburg, The Netherlands. Am. J. Epidemiol. 118: 514–525.
89. Gorelick PB (1987) Alcohol and stroke. Stroke 18: 268–271.
90. Gill JS, Zezulka AV, Shipley MJ, Gill SK and Beevers DG (1986) Stroke and alcohol consumption. N. Engl. J. Med. 315: 1041–1046.
91. Stampfer MJ, Colditz GA, Willett WC, Speizer FE and Hennekens CH (1988) A prospective study of moderate alcohol consumption and the risk of coronary disease and stroke in women. N. Engl. J. Med. 319: 267–273.
92. Leonberg SC and Elliott FA (1981) Prevention of recurrent stroke. Stroke 12: 731–735.
93. Furberg CD, Cutler JA and MacMahon SW (1988) Prevention of stroke: Principles of clinical trials. In: Vinken PJ, Bruyn GW and Klawans HL (eds.) Handbook of clinical neurology, vol. 53, revised series vol. 9, Toole JF (co-ed.). Elsevier Science Publishers, Amsterdam, pp. 459–467.
94. Hypertension Detection and Follow-up Program Cooperative Group (1982) Five year findings of the hypertension detection and follow-up program. III. Reduction in stroke incidence among persons with high blood pressure. J.A.M.A. 247: 633–638.
95. UK-TIA Study Group (1988) United Kingdom transient ischaemic attack (UK-TIA) aspirin trial: Interim results. Br. Med. J. 296: 316–320.
96. Antiplatelet Trialists' Collaboration (1988) Secondary prevention of vascular disease by prolonged antiplatelet treatment. Br. Med. J. 296: 320–331.
97. EC/IC Bypass Study Group (1985) Failure of extracranial-intracranial arterial bypass to reduce the risk of ischaemic stroke: Results of an international randomised trial. N. Engl. J. Med. 313: 1191–1200.
98. Sundt TM (1987) Was the international randomised trial of extracranial-intracranial arterial bypass representative of the population at risk? N. Engl. J. Med. 316: 814–816.
99. Warlow C (1984) Carotid endarterectomy: Does it work? Stroke 15: 1068-1076.
100. Callow AD, Caplan LR, Correll JW, Fields WS, Mohr JP, Moore WS, Robertson JT and Toole JF (1988) Carotid endarterectomy: What is its current status? Am. J. Med. 85: 835–838.

Sudden cerebral arterial occlusion

Hiroshi Mochizuki, Muneshige Tobita and Kyuya Kogure
Department of Neurology, Institute of Brain Diseases, Tohoku University, School of Medicine, 1-1 Seiryo-machi, Aoba-ku, Sendai, Japan 980

Introduction

The human brain requires an uninterrupted supply of glucose and oxygen. Every minute, the brain consumes 100 mg of glucose and 50 ml of oxygen by the way of 70–80 ml/100 g dry-weight/min of arterial supply. Fifteen to 20% of total cardiac output is allocated to the brain in resting state.

When arterial supply is suddenly stopped, the brain cannot function after a few minutes, because of low store of glucose, oxygen and other nutrients in the brain parenchyme.

Many conditions, such as thrombosis, embolism, arteritis and others, produce 'sudden cerebral arterial occlusion'. In this paper, we discuss the mechanism of ischemic brain damage following sudden arterial occlusion and the haemorrheological factors as the risk of sudden arterial occlusion.

Post-ischemic death of selectively vulnerable brain cells

Current studies have revealed that ischaemia-induced death of brain cells are caused by two different mechanisms: 'energy failure' and 'membrane perturbation' [1]. The necrotic locus produced by the former consists of dead neurons, glial cells, and capillary blood vessels, and the necrotising process is accompanied by brain oedema. In contrast, the latter results in neuronal death only in the selectively vulnerable neurons without brain oedema; this feature has been previously described as 'delayed neuronal death' by Kirino et al. [2].

The process of ischaemia-induced neuronal necrosis has been interpreted by postulating; 1) stage of acidosis; 2) stage of energy crisis; 3) stage of disintegration and, 4) stage of autolysis. However, the assumption of energy failure [3] as the cause of cell death in ischaemia cannot account for the mechanism of delayed neuronal necrosis. Our present knowledge of delayed neuronal necrosis can be summarised thus; 1) this form of cell death intervenes suddenly, despite normal blood flow, normal energy state, and normal homeostasis; 2) however, this only occurs in the neurons which receive glutamatergic fibers [4]; 3) the post-ischemic abnormal excitatory state of the cell continues until cell death occurs [5] and, 4) the dying cell will have irretrievably lost its capacity to synthesise protein [6,7].

Let us try and put the above aspects of the ischaemia-induced disorders together in a coherent account that does not contradict any of the experimental evidence. In this context, there has first been an attempt to determine by simulation on a simple model what happens under ischaemia-induced acidosis and energy failure. The reactions arising are as follows: 1) With the onset of ischaemia, the H^+ ion concentration in the cell increases; 2) Some of the H^+ ions are released under the action of the H^+-Na^+ antiport while Na^+ ions will enter the cell. During ischaemia, however, the Na^+ ion pump does not operate as a result of energy failure; 3) The intracellular Na^+ concentration will rise with depolarisation of the cell membrane; 4) As a result, the potential difference-dependent Ca^{2+} channels in the cell membrane will open (voltage-dependent gate opening) so that Ca^{2+} ions will flow into the cell; 5) Due to the energy failure which has occurred, the Ca^{2+} ion pump is not working so that the Ca^{2+} concentration inside the cell will rise.

The above chain of reactions should occur in all of the brain cells at the ischemic site. Distributed in the cell are a large number of enzymes whose function is dependent on Ca^{2+}. These include many auto-digestive processes, so that they may themselves act as the cause of ischemic cell damage if the above reactions go beyond a certain critical point.

If this happens in the presynaptic cells, the result will be a non-specific, uncontrolled release of neuronal transmitters [8,9]. However, if glutamate is released, a receptor-operated Ca^{2+} gate opening will occur in the post-synaptic membrane, and the infusion of Ca^{2+} ions will result in the local activation of calcium activated neutral protease (CAMP) [10]. The activated CAMP will then act on the structural protein (fodrin actin network) lining the lipid bilayer of the cell membrane, with resulting changes in its shape [11]. When these reactions are intensified in ischaemia, the deformation of the structural protein may go as far as its local decomposition. The molecular mechanism of the receptor operated Ca^{2+} gate opening is not yet understood. In case of in vivo experiments, intracellular Ca^{2+} level rises markedly within a few seconds after application of glutamate [12], but the exact speed of Ca^{2+} accumulation in well-buffered brain cells in vivo is not known. Our experiment on the rat hippocampus utilising a particle-induced X-ray emission (PIXE) method indicated that the Ca content of the hippocampus increased 30 min after 20 min global ischaemia [13]. The data in Table 1 show normalisation of Ca content in the hippocampus 2 h after recirculation, but the Zn and Ni values, which are important divalents for the maintenance of Ca^{2+} homeostasis, appear far from the control. A deduction from this is that the vulnerable neurons in the brain lost calcium homeostasis as early as 30 min after being affected by a lethal ischemic insult.

On the whole, the results of our experiment [14] strongly indicate that inositol-containing phospholipids are first degraded by phospholipase C immediately after the decrease of phosphorylation potential, at the same time 1,2-diacyl-glycerol (1,2-DG) and inositol-1,4,5 triphosphate (IP3) are produced, followed by libera-

Table 1. Post-ischemic changes in the concentration of various elements in the rat hippocampus

	Ca	Zn	Ni
Controls (n = 5)	66.26 ± 8.22	77.69 ± 3.15	3.51 ± 0.45
20 min ischaemia + 30 min reperfusion (n = 5)	97.97 ± 17.18[a]	94.14 ± 8.62[a]	1.14 ± 0.73[b]
20 min ischaemia + 2 h reperfusion (n = 5)	67.08 ± 10.31	86.82 ± 6.42[a]	0.67 ± 0.34[b]

Values are means ± SD (μg/g dry weight); [a]$P < 0.05$; [b]$P < 0.01$ (Student's t-test) as compared to the control.

tion of arachidonic acid and other FFAs by the DG lipase and monoacylglycerol lipase system. There may also be a possibility that phospholipase A2 is activated in this model after 2 to 5 min of ischaemia.

IP3 can increase cytosolic calcium concentration by releasing Ca^{2+} from the intracellular Ca^{2+} store [15] and a part of IP3 is converted by IP3 kinase to IP4, which can potentiate Ca^{2+} influx from extracellular space [16], also resulting in an increase in cytosolic Ca^{2+} activity. The effect of Ca^{2+} upon CANP was discussed above.

In the activation of phospholipases, PI-specific phospholipase C is far more sensitive to the Ca^{2+} concentration than phospholipase A2. Therefore, a specific activation of phospholipase C may occur if an increase in Ca^{2+} activity remains at the lower level. However, a massive influx of Ca^{2+} together with mobilisation of the divalent from its endostore may induce non-specific activation of phospholipases during the early period of post-ischemic reperfusion.

Polyunsaturated fatty acids such as arachidonic acid and docosahexaenoic acid play an important role in maintaining the function of the cell membrane through the ability to control fluidity of the lipid bilayer and to regulate the intramembraneous micro-domain from hydrophobic to hydrophilic condition by changing the molecular conformation from trans to cis or gauche, and vice versa. In this manner, the structural protein lining the lipid bilayer and the bilayer itself are both eventually broken down so that the cell membrane is no longer capable of acting as the cell's physiological base, with irreversible perforation of the membrane. The term 'perturbational gate opening' has been proposed to describe the process of cell membrane perforation.

With the cell membrane thus perforated, the cell will not be able to sustain homeostasis if the ischemic condition continues and the eventual result will be the breakdown of the internal cell structure (osmotic effect with energy failure) and cell death (intra-ischemic necrosis). If, however, this process is not allowed to proceed as far as this, and the cell is reperfused with blood before its ultimate breakdown, the mitochondria will resume respiration and the electrolyte pump will be reactivated to allow the cell to regain homeostasis so that it will survive, at least for a while. However, when an excessively large amount of ATP is used up to operate the electrolyte pump, since the mitochondria cannot work beyond their full capacity, the cell will have no spare capacity for any of the additional functions needed, such as, for example, the biosynthesis of replacement substances. As a result, the cell will not be able to replenish through biosynthesis those aging molecules which at the end of their lives have lost their structural and functional usefulness and need replacement. The natural consequence is that at this juncture the internal structure can no longer support the normal molecular structure and function, so that homeostasis of the cell organisation will again be destroyed, with the cell being doomed to a delayed death. This theory has the advantage that it can explain all phenomena under the broad description of 'delayed neuronal necrosis'. Even the 4 turning points such as acute, maturational, delayed neuronal death, and survival, through which the cells subjected to ischemic attack pass, can all be accounted for on the basis of a single theory whereby a severe ischemic attack will result in an excessive perturbational gate opening so that, even though mitochondrial ATP production may be restored at the resumption of the blood supply, the cell will not be able to recover its internal homeostasis and therefore undergo acute changes resulting in its early breakdown. For cells meeting this fate, it seems as if the breakdown and ultimate death are accelerated by the resumption of the blood flow.

On the basis of the above mechanism, several pharmacoprotective agents are designed for the treatment of cerebral ischaemia (Fig. 1).

All the brain cells that receive glutamatergic fibres are profoundly implicated in the realisation of higher brain functions such as: memory (learning and remembering), emotive expression, spontaneity, and skillfulness. The possibility of preventing ischemic necrosis of these neurons is, therefore, tantamount to having developed a means of preventing the onset of the vascular dementia consequent upon cerebral ischaemia. Thus, it is believed that the clinical application of these discoveries will have a significant social impact.

Clinical haemorheology

From the view point of clinical haemorheology, the nature of artery and blood are two major factors. Atherosclerosis, stenosis, mural thrombi, and occlusion are determining factors in the artery. Although the changes of the artery are difficult to treat, the nature of the blood is treatable in clinical aspect of the stroke.

Many factors determine blood viscosity. The number and nature of the blood cells, including red cells, white cells, and platelets, are important. While haematocrit and platelet aggregability were studied as a risk factor of stroke, plasma viscosity is also important in clinical aspects.

Many investigators [17,18] have reported that blood viscosity and haematocrit are useful indices as risk factor in cerebral infarction. Blood viscosity measured in vitro chiefly depends on haematocrit. Haematocrit is the most important factor of

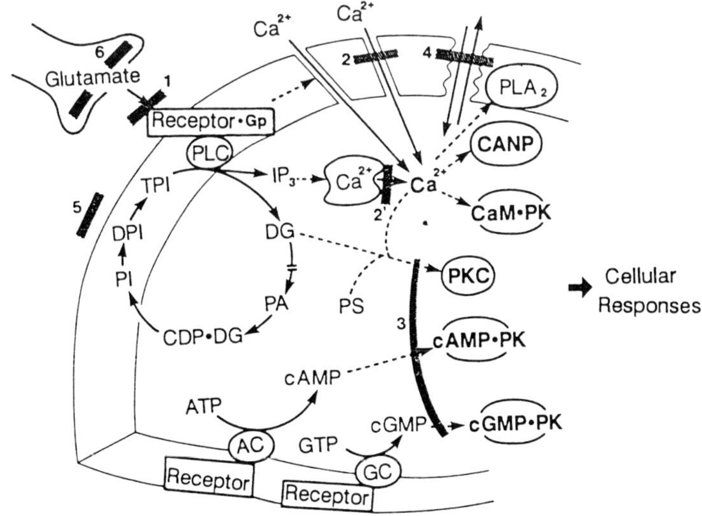

Fig. 1. Mechanism of membrane perturbation and pharmacoprotective agents.
PLA_2: phospholipase A_2
CANP: calcium activated neutral protease
CaM.PK: calmodulin dependent protein kinase
PKC: protein kinase C
PLC: phospholipase C
TPI: triphosphoinositide
DPI: diphosphoinositide
PI: phosphatidylinositol
PI_3: phosphatidylinositol triphosphate
DG: diacyl-glycerol
PA: phosphatidyl acid
PS: phosphatidyl serine
AC: adenylate cyclase
GC: guanilate cyclase
1. Glutamate receptor antagonist
2. Voltage-dependent Ca^{2+} channel blocker
3. Inactivation of kinase, cyclic AMP or cyclic CMP dependent protein kinase
4. Chemical sealing of perturbational gate
5. Activation of inhibitory afferent system
6. Inhibition of excitatory neurotransmitter release

the blood viscosity in the aorta or great artery level, because it relates the 'apparent blood viscosity' and it does not change in the vessels with the diameter of such great artery.

Lipowsky and his colleagues [19] demonstrated that the haematocrit of microvessel decreased to 20% of systemic haematocrit. This means that when systemic haematocrit was 45%, the haematocrit of the microcirculation was 9%. In the small artery or arteriole level, the red cells accumulate in the central axis of the blood flow, and 'plasma sheath' plays an important role. This indicates that plasma viscosity was the determining factor of the blood viscosity in small artery or arteriole levels of microcirculation. In this condition, systemic haematocrit does not affect blood viscosity.

In capillary networks, the diameter of the capillary is smaller than that of the red cell, so the deformability of the red cell is the most determinant factor of the blood viscosity.

These investigations indicate that the determining factors of the blood viscosity vary with the diameter of the vessels. The influence of haematocrit on blood viscosity is most important in the aorta to medium size artery, but plasma viscosity and red cell deformability play the most important role in arterioles and in capillaries, respectively.

An increased plasma viscosity has clinical significance known as a hyperviscosity syndrome; macroglobulinaemia and multiple myeloma with hyper-gamma-globulinaemia in stroke. Fibrinogen, globulins, and other big particles of proteins increase the plasma viscosity. High fibrinogen concentration exacerbates the increased aggregability and decreased deformability of the red cells [20]. On the other hand, albumin may inhibit the fibrinogen-associated decrease in red cell deformability, and high dose content of albumin does not increase the plasma viscosity.

Though the past trials of non-dilutional hypervolaemia with whole blood infusion had failed due to elevated blood viscosity and cellular aggregation [21], by haemorrheological aspects, the treatment with dilutional hypervolaemia has benefits. The dilutional hypervolaemia with decreasing haematocrit, increasing plasma volume, and infusing colloidal plasma expander make blood and plasma viscosity decrease, and red cell aggregability and deformability improve. A favourable relative oxygen transport capacity occurs as haematocrit is lowered to approximately 33% [22]. Wood et al. [23] reported that reduction of haematocrit by venesection had the effect of elevating oxygen transport to the brain in patients with high haematocrit. Wood also reported that hypervolaemic haemodilution improved the regional cerebral blood flow and electroencephalographic monitoring. Their study method was consistent with intravenous colloidal plasma expander infusion and venesection if base line haematocrit was high [24].

We now try the dilutional hypervolemia with the component blood transfusion technique to reduce the haematocrit instead of venesection. We draw the red cell with component collection by component apheresis system, and return plasma to patients with plasma expander such as low-molecular-weight dextran, hydroxyethylated starch, and albumin. In this way, we can reduce the haematocrit, blood viscosity, and plasma viscosity. By this method, we can also expect the improvements of red cell aggregability and deformability, and platelet aggregability and because of preserving the albumin content.

References

1. Kogure K (1980) Biochemistry of intra-ischemic and post-ischemic brain injury. Neurol. Surg. 8: 313–329.
2. Kirino T (1982) Delayed neuronal death in the gerbil hippocampus following ischemia. Brain Res. 239: 57–69.
3. Duffy TE, Nelson SR and Lowry OH (1972) Cerebral carbohydrate metabolism during acute hypoxia and recovery. J. Neurochem. 19: 959–977.
4. Wieloch T (1985) Neurochemical correlates to selective neuronal vulnerability. Progr. Brain Res. 63: 69–85.
5. Suzuki R, Yamaguchi T, Choh-Luh Li and Klatzo I (1983) The effect of 5-min ischemia in mongolian gerbils: II, Changes of spontaneous neuronal activity in cerebral cortex and CA1 sector of hippocampus. Acta Neuropathol. (Berlin) 60: 217–222.
6. Bodsch W, Takahashi K, Barbier B, Ophoff G and Hossmann K-A (1985) Cerebral proteins and ischemia. Progr. Brain Res. 63: 197–210.
7. Sato H, Kogure K, Tobita M and Izumiyama K (1985) Biochemical evaluation of post-ischemic methionine metabolism in gerbil brain: Basic research for the study of PET. J. Cereb. Blood Flow Metab. 5: 5625–5626.
8. Wurtman RI and Zervas MJ (1974) Monoamine neurotransmitters and the pathophysiology of stroke and central nervous system trauma. J. Neurosurg. 40: 34–36.
9. Kogure K, Scheinberg P, Matsumoto A, Busto R and Reinmuth OM (1975) Catecholamines in experimental brain ischemia. Arch. Neurol. 32: 21–24.
10. Lynch F, Larson J, Kelso S, Barrionueve G and Schottler F (1983) Intracellular injection of EGTA block induction of hippocampal long-term potentiation. Nature 305: 719–721.
11. Lynch G and Bawdry M (1984) The biochemistry of memory: A new and specific hypothesis. Science 224: 1057–1063.
12. Kudo Y and Ogura A (1986) Glutamate-induced increase in intracellular Ca^{2+}+ concentration in isolated hippocampal neurones. Br. J. Pharmacol. 89: 191–198.
13. Tsuda T, Kogure K, Ishii K and Orihara H (1990) Post-ischemic changes of calcium and endogenous antagonist in the rat hippocampus studied by proton induced X-ray emission analysis. Brain Res. (in press).
14. Abe K, Kogure K, Yamamoto H, Imazawa M and Miyamoto K (1987) Mechanism of arachidonic acid liberation during ischemia in gerbil cortex. J. Neurochem. 48: 503–509.
15. Berridge MJ and Irvine RF (1984) Inositol triphosphate, a novel second messenger in cellular signal transduction. Nature 312: 315–321.
16. Irvine RF, Letcher AJ, Heslop JP and Berridge MJ (1986) The inositol tris/tetrakisphosphate pathway-demonstration of Ins(1,4,5) P_3 3-kinase activity in animal tissues. Nature 320: 631–634.
17. Grotta J, Ackerman R, Correia J, Fallick G and Chang J (1982) Whole blood viscosity parameter and cerebral blood flow. Stroke 13: 296–301.
18. Tohgi H, Yamanouchi H, Murakami M and Kameyama M (1978) Importance of the hematocrit as risk factor in cerebral infarction. Stroke 9: 369–374.
19. Lipowsky HH, Usami S and Chien S (1980) In vivo measurement of 'Apparent viscosity' and microvessel hematocrit in the mesentery of the cat. Microvascul. Res. 19: 297–319.
20. Sakuta S (1981) Blood filterability in cerebrovascular disorders, with special reference to erythrocyte deformability and ATP. Stroke 12: 824.
21. Sundt TM, Waltz AG and Sayre GE (1967) Experimental cerebral infarction: Modification by treatment with hemodiluting, hemoconcentrating, and dehydrating agents. J. Neurosurg. 26: 46.
22. Hint H (1968) The pharmacology of dextran and the physiological background for the clinical use of Rheochromadex and Macrodex. Acta Anaesthesiol. Belg. 19: 119.
23. Wood JH, Polyzoidis KS, Epsein CM et al. (1984) Quantitative EEG alternations after isovolemic hemodilutional augmentation of cerebral blood flow in stroke patients. Neurology (Cleveland) 34: 764.
24. Wood JH and Kee DB (1986) Clinical rheology of stroke and hemodilution. In: Barnett HJM, Mohr JP, Stein BM and Yatsu FM (eds.) Stroke: Pathophysiology, Diagnosis and Management. Churchill Livingston, New York, pp. 97–108.

Treatment of acute cerebral ischemia by colloid solutions

Alexander Hartmann, Hans Lagreze, Karl Broich and Miriam Fric
Neurologische Universitätsklinik, 5300 Bonn 1, FRG

Acute cerebral ischemia as TIA, PRIND or complete infarction is due to sudden interruption of cerebral blood flow (CBF) to a limited area. Complete cessation of blood circulation to the whole brain (following cardiac arrest) is tolerated well if lasting only for a short period (seconds to few minutes). Partial ischemia to localized regions is tolerated less well and might result in infarction. This is due to collaterals or residual flow, both of which allow secondary metabolic processes leading to: (1) Anaerobic production of lactate with vasoparalysis; (2) Arachidonic acid production with disturbances of the balance between the vasoconstricting Thromboxane A2 and the vasodilating Prostaglandin I2 (Prostaglandin); (3) Free radicals with destruction of cells and blood brain barrier; (4) Intracellular accumulation and sequestration of Calcium-ions with destruction of mitochondria and eventually cell death; (5) Development of (first) cytotoxic and (later) vasogenic brain edema, which impairs oxygen diffusion and cell metabolism.

Since autoregulation is disturbed further on tissue perfusion follows perfusion pressure passively. Increase of intracranial pressure (ICP) due to vasogenic edema or reduction of arterial pressure might then impair the already reduced CBF and favor spread of infarction. Consequently arterial blood pressure should not be too low to prevent increase of infarct size, and not too high to avoid provocation of brain edema by pressing plasma through the destructed blood brain barrier. It seems worthwhile to keep the mean arterial pressure at about 110–130 mmHg.

The brain tissue tries to compensate for the reduced CBF by elevated extraction of oxygen from the arterial blood. For a short period (a few hours) this might keep up the metabolic rate of oxygen and prevent definite infarction. However, after that oxygen extraction falls and altered flow (decreased or increased due to the lactic acidosis with reduction of pH), decreased oxygen extraction and decreased oxygen metabolism mark the beginning of final infarction. At this time any further achievement of improved flow seems to be futile. Any therapeutic manoeuvres which aim at normalizing flow must start before oxygen extraction falls and before lactacidotic hyperemia occurs. Fortunately the regional pattern varies even within one region of ischemia giving hope for an eventual beneficial effect of CBF improvement even at a later state.

The infarct core which can almost never be influenced except by very early restoration of flow (thrombolysis with urokinase, streptokinase or tPA) is surrounded by the so-called penumbra where the tissue perfusion is reduced and might be on the point of developing normal function or characteristics of an infarct. The penumbra itself is surrounded by a hyperemic zone which does not benefit from further flow increase.

Since tissue function does depend on the actual flow (flow threshold theory) it seems worthwhile to normalize flow at a very early stage. This should not be done by increasing systemic pressure since this affects all tissues and not only the tissue with reduced flow. Vasodilatation (by CO_2, vasodilating agents) primarily affects normally perfused tissue and therefore is not of benefit.

Since intravascular flow characteristics depend on the actual flow it should be considered whether increase of CBF by altering rheologic parameters might result in improved tissue function.

With decrease of CBF, shear stress increases and results in decrease of shear rate. Since hematocrit is one of the major factors influencing shear stress it has been speculated that decrease of hematocrit might improve flow. This principle of hemodilution has been tried in several studies in acute stroke cases. Since the results are not uniform the studies will be summarized briefly. Thereafter the substances used for hemodilution will be described and after that our own data which indicate that CBF can be increased by hemodilution will be presented.

Haemodilution studies

Gilroy et al. [1] have observed a significant improvement of patients with ischemic stroke following three days hypervolemic demodilution with dextran. The study was done prospectively and randomized and dextran was compared to glucose. In the dextran-group mortality was 4% and in the glucose-group 15%.

Spudis et al. [2] have performed a similar study, again with three days treatment with dextran, and observed a 20% mortality in the dextran-group but only a 10% mortality in the glucose-group. In this prospective randomized study, neurological improvement in the surviving patients was better with dextran than with glucose.

In 1976 Matthews et al. [3] reported on a prospective randomized study in which either dextran or glucose were given for three days to patients with ischemic stroke. During hospitalization mortality in the dextran-group was lower than in the glucose group whereas there was no significant difference between both groups with respect to neurologic improvement in the surviving patients.

The alteration of hematocrit during haemodilution was not reported in any of these three studies.

Since development of brain edema contributes significantly to the fate of the ischemic tissue, Kaste et al. [4] combined in a double blind, prospective randomized study dextran with dexamethasone, and did not observe a significant difference between the treated and the control-group with respect to the neurological condition.

However, Matthew et al. [5] described a significant neurologic improvement by administration of the haemodiluting agent glycerol in patients with ischemic stroke. The study was performed double blind controlled, prospectively and randomized. Since glycerol has a significant effect on brain edemia a beneficial effect cannot be attributed solely to the haemodiluting action.

However, all studies performed until the end of the 70s were not convincing enough to introduce hypervolemic haemodilution as a routine measure in patients with ischemic stroke. Therefore Strano et al. [6] performed an open controlled randomized prospective study using a combination of venesection and early infusion of dextran and observed a reduction of the mortality from 8 to 2% (compared to the untreated control-group) and an improvement of the neurologic score from 64 to 85%. In this study only patients, whose symptoms did not last longer than 48 h were included in the protocol. There was no difference with respect to the number of patients, mean age, sex distribution or previous medical history. In the haemodiluted group, hematocrit was reduced from 43 to 37% within two days and was maintained until the 10th day. There was only a slight reduction of hematocrit in the control group from 43 to 41%. Three months after the stroke had occurred 10% of the haemodiluted and 28% of the control patients had to be treated in the hospital or a nursing home. Eight percent of the survivors in the treated group and 36% of the survivors in the control group were severely impaired (bedridden or confined to a wheelchair).

However, the beneficial effects could not be repeated by a multicenter study by the same authors [7]. Again, the study was done open controlled (dextran versus electrolyte solution) prospectively and randomized. In 183 patients of the dextran group haematocrit was reduced from 44 to 37%, and there was no significant alteration of the haematocrit in the control group. Three months after stroke onset the fatality rate was 16% in the dextran- and 12% in the control-group. There was no significant difference in the neurologic scores of both groups. This protocol of mixed hypervolemic and isovolemic haemodilution led to myocardial infarction or left ventricular failure in 13 haemodiluted and 5 control patients. With respect to subgroup analysis the authors did not find any significant difference between haemodiluted and control patients with respect to the age of the stroke (12 to 48 hours), the severity of neurologic disability and the entrance into the study, or the haematocrit.

This important study does not indicate a beneficial effect of haemodilution in patients with ischemic stroke. In addition it should be noted, that the mortality in haemodiluted patients with a deep localized brain infarct (basalganglia) was higher than in control patients. However, this study was criticized for several reasons, including the fact that some patients entered the protocol not earlier than 52 h after the symptoms began. Still it must be admitted, that in this protocol the short term administration of dextran for three days combined with an early venesection does not lead to a significant improvement of neurologic condition or a significant reduction of mortality.

A similar conclusion was drawn by the authors of the Italian Acute Stroke Study

Group [8]. However, in this study there are no data available on the infusion mode in the control group. The selection of patients for entering the protocol was rather superficially described and the follow-up data were received by information from the family by telephone.

The first study, which did not use low molecular weight dextran by hydroxyethyl starch was performed by Grotta al. [9] as an open controlled, randomized multicenter study. Hypervolemic haemodilution with hydroxyethyl starch was rather aggressive following the hypothesis, that a high perfusion pressure is one of the most important factors for microcirculation and should be improved significantly with very early fast increase of intravascular volume. However, the study was discontinued after the observation that in the hydroxyethyl starch group (HES) significantly more patients died due to brain edema. Incidentally severe strokes were distributed more often in the HES group than in the control group and these patients died more often following the hypervolemic haemodilution. With respect to subgroup analysis in the total of 38 patients a trend of beneficial effect of haemodilution with HES was observed in those patients who entered the protocol within 12 h or where haematocrit reduction was very strong. From this study it must be concluded that patients with early signs of ischemic brain edema should not be treated with hypervolemic haemodilution and that there could be a positive trend in improving mortality and neurologic symptoms if haemodilution in patients without brain edema is started very early and leads to a significant reduction of the haematocrit.

The studies using dextran or a hydroxyethyl starch, performed in the 80s, were not done on a blind basis. This, however, seems to be difficult due to the colloid structure and appearance of the haemodiluting solutions, the colour of the agents and the fact that observation of the haematocrit allows a definite decision, whether the patient is treated with normal saline or colloid solution.

A double blind controlled, randomized, prospective, multicenter study in patients with ischemic stroke was done with pentoxyfilline [10]. In this protocol patients were treated with placebo or with 1200 mg pentoxyfilline intravenously by oral administration. There was a significant improvement of mortality and neurologic outcome within the first three days (during the intravenous administration of the substance) in the treated group compared to the control group and persistence of the beneficial effect in the following days until the 28th day. In our opinion this study indicates that early treatment of patients with ischemic stroke with intravenous administration of pentoxyfilline might be of significant benefit to the patients. The consequence from the observation, that the significance after the third day was altered to a positive trend should be that intravenous administration should be prolonged and not stopped after the third day of treatment. Since this is the first study which evaluated the course of the outcome and mortality in patients with ischemic stroke on a multicenter, double blind, randomized, prospective basis, the importance of this protocol should not be discarded.

The conclusion from all studies referred to in this overview is that both beneficial and negative results have been described with dextran, that one study using hydroxyethyl starch led to negative results in patients with developing brain edema but beneficial effects in patients without brain edema and early start of therapy or significant reduction of haematocrit and that in patients with ischemic stroke even Pentoxyfilline might result in beneficial effects if the substance is given intravenously.

A further important study has been published by Korosue et al. [11]. In this protocol isovolemic haemodilution with venesection and administration of fresh plasma led to the reduction of the haematocrit by 27% and an increase in the cardiac output without significant alteration in perfusion pressure. Despite this lack of increased perfusion pressure, regional cerebral blood flow increased by 30% in the ischemic area of the middle cerebral artery which was related inversely to the haematocrit and the whole blood viscosity. At the same time a significant improvement in the neurologic condition was observed. This study indicates that even without increases of perfusion pressure cerebral blood flow might be improved leading to clinically beneficial effects.

The availability of dextran, hydroxyethyl starch, pentoxifylline or fresh plasma in combination with venesection does not facilitate the decision of which substance should be used for haemodilution.

Haemodiluting agents

Low molecular weight dextran

It is a strong hyperoncotic agent which, using the solution with a mean molecular weight of 40,000 – might lead to an increase of plasma viscosity if infused over several days. This is due to the fact that high molecular particles in the solution are not excreted fast enough by the kidney. In patients with diabetes, dextran therapy might lead to acute renal failure. This is partially due to the increase of urinary viscosity by dextran [12]. Dextran might lead to anaphylactoid reactions which might be reduced by the infusion of dextran-haptens [13,14] prior to the start of the dextran infusion. The avoidance of anaphylactoid reactions, however, by the use of haptens is not complete [15]. The volume effect of dextran 40 is about 100% which should be taken into account if the patient suffers from cardiac insufficiency [16]. In addition to the increase of plasma viscosity dextran 40 might increase red cell aggregation. The clinical effect by this factor which might impair microcirculation is not clear [17].

Hydroxyethyl starch

The volume effect of low molecular starch solutions like hydroxyethyl starch with a mean molecular weight of 40,000 is less than that of Dextran 40. The increase of plasma volume lasts for about three hours [18]. In contrast to Dextran 40 there is a reduction of plasma viscosity. The excretion from the body of the high molecular hydroxyethyl starch (mean molecular weight of 200,000) is rather fast in the first days but after that slower than in Dextran 40 [19]. HES might provoke anaphylactoid reactions, the frequency is not clear. There is no way to prevent these anaphylactoid reactions by any prophylactic measures. In patients with long time dialysis, development of ascites has been described following hepatic disposition of HES [20].

Pentoxifylline

Pentoxifylline leads only to a minor reduction of haematocrit. Its advantage is the improvement of microcirculation by increase of red cell filterability (red cell deformability), reduction of plasma viscosity and decrease of red cell and platelet aggregation. Tissue oxygenation is improved [21,22].

Haemodilution and cerebral blood flow

The equation of Hagen-Poisseuille, which is partially applicable to cerebral vessels with their constantly changing diameter indicates that cerebral blood flow (CBF) depends on perfusion pressure, vascular resistance, the length of the vessel and the blood viscosity. With increase of haematocrit and concentration of high molecular protein (Fibrinogen) blood viscosity rises [23]. Furthermore, microcirculation depends on the capability of the red cells to alter for passage of small caliber capillaries. With increase of haematocrit, CBF decreases to compensate for the increased number of transported oxygen-carrying particles. This results in a constant oxygen consumption. Patients with polyglobulia therefore have a decreased blood flow in the presence of constant oxygen extraction. On the other side patients with anemia present with increased tissue perfusion to keep the oxygen consumption constant [24,25].

If vascular obstruction leads to acute reduction of CBF (acute ischemic stroke) this cannot be compensated for by autoregulatory vasodilatation and unlimited increase of oxygen extraction. Under these circumstances oxygen consumption is reduced and results in ischemic stroke. Since normal whole blood viscosity depends on sufficient tissue perfusion reduction of CBF provokes further increase of viscosity, which then again results in another drop of tissue perfusion [26]. It has been shown by several studies that increase of viscosity due to high haematocrit is associated with an increased risk of brain infarction [27,28].

Therefore it seems worthwhile to increase CBF in the presence of primary cerebral ischemia by reduction of whole blood viscosity for the sake of tissue perfusion. This cannot be done by pure venesection with removal of blood and red cells since this does not result in reduction of whole blood viscosity. However, venesection plus compensation for the drawn volume by infusion of colloid infusions (isovolemic haemodilution) or infusion of colloid solutions like molecular weight dextran, hydroxyethyl starch or albumine (hypervolemic haemodilution) results in decrease of whole blood viscosity and therefore should increase the tissue perfusion.

As early as 1969 Gottstein and Held showed that infusion of 10% low molecular weight dextran (LMWD) decreases haematocrit and increases CBF with concomitant slight increase of oxygen consumption [29]. After several authors could prove the dependency of cerebral blood flow on haematocrit and whole blood viscosity [30–33] an attempt was made to improve decreased tissue perfusion in the presence of brain infarction by reduction of physiologic whole blood viscosity. Experimental studies have shown that hypervolemic haemodilution by autologous plasma or LMWD might improve tissue perfusion in animals with acute ischemia [34,35] and at the same time it was shown that by these measures infarct size might be reduced significantly [36]. Wood et al. observed that tissue perfusion is more marked in areas with low flow or decreased shear rate and less increased in normally perfused tissue [37]. This is completely in agreement with our physiologic understanding and was supported by identical results in patients with ischemic stroke, where hydroxyethyl starch with subsequent reduction of haematocrit increases flow in the ischemic tissue [38]. Even with mannitol, which leads to some moderate haemodilution but primarily acts as tissue water reducing agent, blood flow increases more in the ischemic than in other areas [39]. Observation by others [40] did not evaluate the effect of haemodilution on primary ischemic tissue but only the effect of venesection in cats under mild shock condition. These results are not relevant to the question of whether haemodilution in ischemic stroke is of more benefit to the ischemic or the normally perfused tissue.

Controversial arguments have been presented by Brown and Marshall [41]. They described a lack of correlation between viscosity and blood flow and a significant dependency of tissue perfusion on arterial oxygen content. However, these results have been obtained in patients with solely paraproteinemia and therefore normal perfusion pressure.

Own studies in baboons focused on the question whether different haemodiluting agents influence rheological parameters in a different way [35]. It could be shown that hypervolemic haemodilutions under physiological state with hydroxyethyl starch lead to slight reduction of plasma viscosity and slight reduction of haematocrit. The consequence was a significant increase of CBF. With infusion of LMWD, plasma viscosity increased and haematocrit decreased significantly, resulting in no change of CBF. With infusion of normal saline, plasma viscosity and CBF remained constant despite slight reduction of haematocrit from 40 to 37%. There was no difference between the three groups with respect to changes of blood pressure, heart rate, central venous pressure and blood gases. We do not have any definite explanation why LMWD did not increase tissue perfusion under these conditions of physiologic state. We cannot exclude a negative effect of increased plasma viscosity on microcirculation. However, the significant reduction of hematocrit from 39 to 30% should usually increase flow even with infusion of dextran.

Quite different results have been observed in patients suffering from acute ischemic stroke. The following protocol has been performed:

Table 1. Hemodynamic parameters in baboons with infarction

		maBP	CVP	$PaCO_2$	HR	HCT
SS	D	98.2/5.8	4.2/0.4	39.2/2.1	88/12	41.4/2.3
CBF1	C	104.6/4.8	3.2/0.6	40.1/1.4	92/17	40.7/2.0
AR	D	78.4/4.3	3.5/0.2	38.2/3.0	96/18	41.0/2.2
	C	80.2/7.5	2.9/1.8	39.7/3.1	96/18	39.6/3.1
CO2-	D	3.2/0.3	5.3/1.3		88/10	41.3/2.8
RF	C	3.0/0.6	4.2/1.9		92/8	40.9/2.0
CBF2	D	97.6/6.8	4.4/2.7	40.1/3.7	84/12	41.8/2.2
	C	101.2/5.0	3.6/0.9	39.6/2.0	92/12	39.4/2.7
CBF3	D	99.2/4.6	6.1/0.9	41.3/3.4	98/15	37.2/2.5
	C	100.3/3.6	3.9/1.8	38.8/2.7	98/6	37.0/1.6
CBF4	D	104.2/6.9	7.2/1.3	40.8/1.9	88/13	36.8/2.0
	C	104.3/3.8	3.3/0.9	40.5/2.3	84/16	39.5/3.5

SS, AR, and CO2-RF are measurment during pre-clip condition; CBF 2 was done right after positioning of the MCA-clip; CBF 3 was measured after end of infusion and CBF 4 60 after end of infusion; D = group with infusion of low molecular weight dextrane; C = control group (infusion of normal saline).

maBP = mean arterial blood pressure (mmHg); CVP = central venous pressure (mmHg); PaCO2 = arterial CO2 partial pressure (mmHg); HR = heart rate (per min).

In patients with acute ischemic stroke in supratentorial tissue in whom CBF studies could be performed within 24 h after onset of symptoms randomized distribution to the following three groups have been performed:

a) control group: daily treatment with 500 ml of normal saline or 5% glucose in addition to normal fluid.
b) HES group: daily infusion of 10% hydroxyethyl starch 200,000, 500 ml/day for 7 days.
c) LMWD group: daily infusion of 10% low molecular weight dextran, 500 ml for 7 days.

CBF has been measured on day 1 before the infusion, on the following day and on the 7th day (the last day of infusion).

In the control group there was no significant change of CBF in the non-ischemic, contralateral hemisphere, but a slight decrease of mean CBF from day 1 to day 2.

In the HES group blood flow increased significantly in both hemispheres from day 1 to day 2 and from there to day 7.

The same has been shown for the LMWD group. Despite treatment for seven days a normalization of blood flow was only observed in the contralateral hemisphere but not in the ischemic hemispheres.

In this protocol there was no difference between the HES and LMWD groups. Again, it was noted, that hypoxemic tissue benefited significantly more from haemodilution than normally perfused tissue. This trend was observed for the control group as well but more pronounced in patients treated with oncotic agents [30].

These results point to an improvement of tissue perfusion under ischemic conditions. This observation does not indicate whether metabolism benefits from increase of CBF. Since even the natural course of CBF during ischemic infarction involves naturally occurring hyperemia (following development of lactic acidosis) one should keep in mind, that haemodilution is contraindicated in the state of hyperemia. Furthermore, the territorial alteration of flow with the ischemic core (which is untreatable), the penumbra (with reduced flow and increased oxygen extraction fraction), and the hyperemic neighbouring tissue prohibits a routine haemodilution in patients with ischemic stroke. From the pathophysiologic point of view haemodilution should aim only at improving flow in the penumbra and therefore these and other measures of improving flow in patients with ischemic stroke should be correlated thoroughly to the flow data obtained with routine measurement of blood flow. In our opinion it is careless to treat patients with ischemic stroke without repeated routine measurement of cerebral blood flow.

The beneficial and clinical effects of one multicenter study with pentoxifylline-treatment in acute ischemic stroke have not been correlated to blood flow measurements. Our own observations point to an improvement of flow in patients with chronic vascular disease [42]. The pronounced effect on ischemic tissue again points to a selected effect of rheological parameters on local tissue flow. Pilot observations in patients with acute stroke again indicate, that 900 mg pentoxifylline/day administered intravenously, over a period of 7 days might lead to increase of CBF.

References

1. Gilroy JM, Barnhart J and Meyer JS (1969) J. Amer. Med. Ass. 210: 293–298.
2. Spudis EV, De la Torre E and Pikula, L (1973) Stroke 4: 895–897.
3. Matthews WB, Oxbury JM, Grainger KMR and Greenhall RCD (1976) Brain 99: 193–306.
4. Kaste M, Fogelholm R and Waltimo O (1976) Br. Med. J. 2: 1409–1410.
5. Mathew NM, Meyer JS, Rivera V, Charney JS and Hartmann A (1972) Lancet: 1327–1329.
6. Strand T, Asplund K, Eriksson S, Hagge E, Lithner F and Wester PO (1984) Stroke 15: 980–989.
7. Asplund K (1989) Acta Neurol Scand, Suppl. 172: 22–30.
8. Italian Acute Stroke Study Group (1988) Lancet I: 318–321.
9. Grotta JC (1987) Stroke 18: 689–690.
10. Hsu CY, Norris JW, Hogan EL et al. (1988) Stroke 19: 716–722.
11. Korosue K, Ishida K, Matsuoka H, Nagao T, Tamaki N and Matsumoto S (1988) Neurosurgery 23: 148–153.
12. Schneider, Cremer W (1983) Nieren- und Hochdruckkrankheiten 12: 301–305.
13. Bergentz S, Falkheden T and Olson S (1965) Ann. Surg. 161: 582–586.
14. Gruber UF, Allemann U and Wettler H (1982) Schweiz Med. Wschr. 122: 605–612.

15. Laubenthal H, Peter K, Richter W, Kraft D, Selbmann HK and Messmer K (1983) Diagnostik und Intensivtherapie 8: 4–14.
16. Schoning B, Sommer K and Koch H (1984) Anaesth. Intensivth. Notfallmed. 19: 34–37.
17. Kohler H (1978) Intensivbehandlung 3: 138–144.
18. Staedt U, Schwarz M and Heene DL (1986) Med. Welt I: 660–663.
19. Kortilla K, Growhn P, Gordin A, Sundberg S, Salo H, Nissinen E and Mattila MAK (1984) J. Clin. Pharmacol. 24: 273–282.
20. Kohler H, Zschiedrich H, Linfante A, Appel F, Pitz H and Clasen R (1982) Klin. Wschr. 60: 293–301.
21. Pfeifer U, Kult J and Forster H (1984) Klin. Wschr. 62: 862–866.
22. Muller R (1979) J. Med. 10: 307–318.
23. Ehrly (1983) Am. Vasc. Med. 1: 175–179.
24. Gottstein U (1965) Med. Welt 15: 715–726.
25. Gottstein U (1969) Verh. Dtsch. Ges. Inn. Med. 75: 957–965.
26. Schmid Schonbein H (1981) In: Microcirculation. Effrons RM, Schmid-Schonbein H, Ditzel J, (eds.) Academic Press, New York, pp. 249–261.
27. Thomas DJ (1982) Stroke 13: 285–287.
28. Dawber TR (1980) Harvard University Press, Cambridge MA.
29. Gottstein U and Held K (1969) Dtsch. Med. Wschr. 94: 522–526.
30. Hartmann A, Tusda Y and Lagreze H (1987) J. Neurol. 235: 34–38.
31. Vorstrup S, Andersen A, Juhler M, Brun B and Boysen G (1986) Acta. Neurol. Scand. 73: 530–531.
32. Wood HY, Polyzoidis KS, Epstein CM, Gibby GL and Tindall GT (1983) J. Cereb. Blod. Flow Metab. 3: 588–589.
33. Herrschaft H (1984) Beitr. Anaesth. Intensivmed. 3: 106–125.
34. Wood JH, Simeone FA, Fink EA and Golden MA (1984) Neurology 34: 24–29.
35. Tsuda Y, Hartmann A, Weiand J and Solymosi L (1987) J. Neurol. Sci. 82: 171–180.
36. Sundt Tm, Waltz AC and Sayre GP (1967) J. Neurosurg. 26: 46–56.
37. Wood JH, Simeone FA, Snyder LL, Fink EA and Golden MA (1981) J. Cereb. Blood Flow. Metab., Suppl. 1: 178–179.
38. Adams RJ, Nichols FT, Highes D and Hill S (1987) In: Cerebral Ischemia and Hemorheology. Hartmann A, Kuschinsky W (eds.) Springer, Berlin, Heidelberg, New York, pp. 416–422.
39. Muizellar JP, Wei EP, Kontos HA and Becker DP (1986) Stroke 17: 44–48.
40. Kummer VR, Scharf R, Back T, Reich H, Machens HG and Wildemann B (1987) Stroke 19: 594–597.
41. Brown MM and Marshall J (1982) Br. Med. J. 284: 1733–1736.
42. Hartmann A and Tsuda Y (1988) Angiology 39: 449–457.

Acute intracranial venous thrombosis

J.S. Chopra and S.K. Bansal

Department of Neurology, Postgraduate Institute of Medical Education and Research, Chandigarh, India

Population-based epidemiological work on stroke is sparse from developing countries. The hospital-based observations reveal an increase in prevalence of stroke with age. Cerebrovascular accidents due to intracranial sinus venous thrombosis more often affect young persons. Thrombosis of cerebral sinuses or veins may occur spontaneously without known cause, 'primary', or as a sequelae of focal sepsis following oto-, rhino- or haematogenous infections. Septic thrombosis has become rare in the antibiotic era.

Patients with acute spontaneous thrombosis fall into two groups. The first group is infants in whom thrombosis may occur during a systemic illness such as diarrhoea and dehydration, cachexia, malnutrition, haemotological malignancies and congenital heart disease. The clinical picture may mimic metabolic encephalopathy similar to water intoxication in an infant who has been rehydrated rapidly. In older children predisposing causes are infections and infectious diseases. The second group is adults of whom the majority of cases are females affected during puerperium. Although all types of cerebral venous thrombosis (CVT) are encountered in clinical experience, we will pay more attention to CVT seen in young females especially during puerperium.

Western observers considered this illness a rare occurrence in puerperium, whereas reports from the Indian subcontinent are alarming. Superior sagittal or longitudinal sinus is most frequently involved in isolation and sometimes in combination with other sinuses (transverse, sigmoid, straight or petrosal) or major cerebral veins. Involvement of the deep intracranial venous system is seen more often in children. A case initially labelled 'primary' may be reclassified 'secondary' after its cause becomes apparent in the natural course of the disease. Averback [1] remarked that primary cortical venous thrombosis in young adults is an 'underdiagnosed disease'. He published seven cases of idiopathic nature.

Prevalence

The exact prevalence of this entity remains uncertain particularly in males and children [2,3]. Less severe cases do not prove fatal or the diagnosis is missed. Caroll et al. [4] found that usually one case a year is seen in any large hospital

(1/2500 deliveries). Among Indian women who suffered stroke, 50% were related to pregnancy and puerperium and 95.5% of these were due to CVT [5]. The Registrar General's returns for England and Wales during 1952–1961 revealed an average of 21.7 deaths annually caused by intracranial thrombophlebitis. Infection was a common underlying factor in 39 out of 73 clinical cases of CVT reported by Krayenbuhl [6].

A large series of 38 cases with angiographically proven CVT observed during 1975–1982 has been recently reviewed by Bousser et al. [7]. The authors stressed that the incidence is falsely low as diagnosis of CVT is extremely difficult unless a high degree of clinical suspicion is confirmed with investigations. Gates [8] reported 66 cases collected from teaching hospitals in Australia. In 15 of 29 fatal cases who underwent autopsy the diagnosis of CVT was not suspected before death. Reports from India [9] highlight a higher incidence of up to 4.5 per 1000 obstetric admissions. A total of about 600 cases has been reported so far from India and in the majority the diagnosis was made on clinical grounds. In a series of 80 cases [10] the diagnosis was confirmed in 32 cases at autopsy. In this series 40 were males. Most of them were from poor socioeconomic status and mostly consumed illicit country liquor. The diagnosis of cerebral venous occlusion was missed in 28% of 32 cases amongst the 8500 non-selected medical autopsies in a period of 14 years [11]. In the literature at least 55 cases of CVT have been related to oral contraceptives.

Primary sino-venous thrombosis is even rarer in young males and children. The earlier reports were by Byers and Hess (1933) and Woolf (1955). Cottrill and Kaplan [12] reported 29 patients who had stroke complicating congenital heart disease. Bousser et al. [7] and Chiras et al. [13] have reported cases of variable aetiology, of which 12 were due to Behcet's disease.

Functional anatomy

The cerebral venous system is a valveless, trabeculated (superior sagittal sinus), low pressure system with easy flow alterations. Apart from the inferior sagittal and straight sinuses the dural venous sinuses are rigidly anchored triangular non-collapsible tubes which maintain normal function despite negative intracranial venous pressure. The veins enter the dural sinuses in a direction opposite to the flow of blood minimizing Venturi effect which would otherwise collapse the veins. The deep venous system comprises the basal veins formed by the deep middle cerebral, anterior cerebral and striate veins. These join the internal cerebral veins to form the great vein of Galen. The latter joined by the inferior sagittal sinus form the straight sinus. The vein of Trolard and the vein of Labbe are the largest of numerous anastomotic channels. They provide alternative routes of venous drainage in the event of occlusions of the intracranial veins and sinuses or adversely facilitate spread of infection or thrombus.

Clinical features

Clinically the diagnosis is presumptive. Heterogenous presentation is known and the diagnosis is missed unless supported by a high degree of suspicion and investigations. The signs and symptoms of acute sino-venous occlusions are either due to primary haemorrhagic infarct or its secondary effects. Thrombosis of the deep cortical veins mostly causes dramatic and severe neurological deficit with or without raised intracranial pressure. It may be acute fulminant or slowly progressive.

Headache is generally a presenting symptom. Its intensity usually parallels the severity of cerebral lesion. It is often severe, persistent, does not respond to analgesics and may suggest a neuralgic character. It is caused by raised intracranial pressure or involvement of pain-sensitive walls of venous sinuses. Seizures begin early. All type of seizures are reported [14]. Hemiplegia is common. Cortical paraplegia ensues following involvement of cortical veins of both hemispheres. Headache and motor weakness may become evident following control of seizures and improvement in the sensorium.

Involvement of cranial nerves is rare and if present it is usually due to raised intracranial pressure or cavernous sinus thrombosis. In rapidly fatal cases, neck rigidity, Cheyne stokes respiration and hyperpyrexia may occur within a few hours of presentation. Symptoms due to thrombosis of dural sinuses are usually less dramatic than those of cerebral vein thrombosis and are mostly limited to raised intracranial pressure. Oedema and tenderness over the mastoid may suggest occlusion of sigmoid sinus (Griesinger's sign). The clinical features can be classified into four groups.

1. Commonly observed acute vascular catastrophic stroke, mostly presenting with headache, focal neurological deficit and convulsions.
2. Subacute 'pseudo stroke'-like onset. Majority have papilloedema and need differentiation from cerebral abscess, tumours and tuberculoma.
3. Presentation akin to diffuse encephalopathy.
4. A few patients present as organic brain syndrome and end up with psychiatrists.

The majority of patients fall into the first group. However, invariably clinical presentation other than acute episode under group one are also encountered. In our experience the clinical presentation falls under these four groups irrespective of the aetiological processes encountered in Table 1. Since the majority of cases of CVT are seen during pregnancy and puerperium the following clinical symptomatology forms the basis of classical picture. In our data of 83 cases of CVT 55 cases were related to pregnancy and puerperium. The mean age of presentation was 27 years (14–40) and most of these patients became symptomatic within the first two weeks of puerperium. These patients had poor or no antenatal check up and underwent home deliveries by untrained midwives. Anaemia, multiparity, fluid restriction following delivery and excessive consumption of fat during pregnancy are other factors noted in the majority of such patients. Antepartum sinus venous thrombosis is rare. However, it can occur in any trimester or after abortion [14].

Table 1. Predisposing factors for cerebral venous thrombosis (CVT)

1. Local factors
    - Head trauma
    - Intracranial surgery
    - Facial infections
    - Tuberculous meningitis
    - Neoplasm
    - Neurosyphilis
    - Cerebral vascular malformation
    - Arachnoid cyst
    - Carcinomatous meningitis

2. Systemic diseases
    - Mostly in infants and children
        - Dehydration
        - Neonatal asphyxia
        - Anaemia, malnutrition and Cachexia
        - Congenital cyanotic heart disease
        - Measles, typhoid, bronchopneumonia, pulmonary tuberculosis
        - Suppuration
    - Diabetes mellitus
    - Diabetic ketoacidosis
    - Nephrotic syndrome
    - Hypotension shock
    - Ulcerative colitis
    - Lupus erythematosus
    - Respiratory failure
    - Herpes zoster opthalmaticus
    - Histiocytosis and radiotherapy
    - Behcet's syndrome
    - Budd Chiari syndrome
    - Congestive cardiac failure

3. Haematological disorders
    - Malignancies such as lymphoma, chronic myeloid leukaemia
    - Disseminated intravascular coagulation
    - Polycythaemia, rubra, vera
    - Iron deficiency anaemia
    - Haemolytic uraemic syndrome
    - Anti-thrombin III deficiency
    - Thrombocytopenia
    - Paroxysmal nocturnal haemoglobin urea
    - Sickle cell trait
    - Haemolytic anaemia

4. Pregnancy, puerperium and the contraceptive pills

5. Idiopathic 'primary'

Signs of meningeal irritation are rare and may be due to entry of blood into the subarachnoid space following haemorrhagic infarction. High grade pyrexia not related to infection is possibly due to the thrombotic process itself [4]. Deep leg vein thrombosis seen in about 10% of the cases of puerperal CVT may precede or follow cerebral infarction [5]. Seven out of our 55 cases of puerperal CVT had associated deep leg vein thrombosis.

Other rare clinical features are cortical blindness, persistent hypotension, postural hypotension, hypothermia, hypoglycemia with sweating and akinetic mutism. These result from involvement of the visual cortex and the hypothalamus. Persistent tachycardia seen in the recovery period suggests impending pulmonary infarction and is an ominous sign. Some such patients collapsed during defaecation 2 weeks following discharge from the hospital [15].

The relationship between the duration of contraceptive pill intake and CVT is not clearly established. In most of the reported cases the duration of intake was short.

Byers and Hass (1933), in their collection of 50 cases in infants and children, emphasized that dural sinus thrombosis is one of the causes of hyperpyrexia in early life. At this age superior sagittal sinus thrombosis is usually silent and convulsions are attributed to fever. The scalp vein dilatation with or without scalp oedema may be a useful observation for diagnosis of this condition in children. Other symptoms such as failure to thrive, refusal to feed, vomiting, loss of weight, irritability and alteration in sensorium may favour this diagnosis [7]. Infarction of the diencephalon and basal ganglia may occur and lead to dystonia, tremor or dyskinesia [16].

Pathogenesis

The authors in the past laid stress to the inflammatory changes in the walls of the sinuses since they included septic cases in their material. Infections are still the single common identifiable cause of CVT [8] even in the era of antibiotics. A wide variety of conditions associated with CVT have recently been reported (Table 1). There is no single known factor which can explain the occurrence of such disorder in all the cases. The exact aetiology of primary intracranial venous thrombosis remains obscure. However, many postulates have been made although none is entirely satisfactory.

Anatomical factors

Intracranial sinuses lack the pumping action of the muscles which may promote stasis of the blood in cerebral sinuses. Trabaculations within the sinuses may also be a contributing factor. Occasionally membranous structure dividing the superior sagittal sinus is an additional factor for the frequent involvement of the superior sagittal sinus. An increase in the incidence of CVT during normal or complicated perinatal period has been explained on the basis of increased intra-abdominal pressure during parturition. The suggestion of retrograde venous embolisation from the pelvic veins to intracranial sinuses through valveless vertebral venous channels has not been found plausible.

Hypercoagulable state

It is the most frequently accepted mechanism to explain the occurrence of CVT in the majority of cases. Blood viscosity increases due to reticular cell malignancies, haemolytic uraemic syndrome, haemolytic anaemia, antithrombin III deficiency, sickle cell trait, pregnancy and due to polycythaemia in cyanotic congenital heart disease. There are many other factors which have been shown to increase the coagulability of the blood. It is supported by frequent occurrence of extracerebral thrombosis. The hypercoagulable state has been shown to be caused by a 100% increase in platelet count [6], increase in the platelet adhesiveness [17], hyperfibrinogenaemia [5,18] and a fall in fibrinolytic activity [19]. Plasma fibrinogen levels were significantly increased in 86.6% of puerperal CVT cases [5]. Increase in platelet count has been shown in puerperal CVT when parturition is complicated by postpartum haemorrhage. The peak increase in platelets occurs around the tenth postpartum day. This is the usual time when venous thrombosis manifests. A rise in the serum lipids has also been shown to play a role in the causation of CVT [20]. A statistically significant increase in the alpha and beta lipoprotein, triglycerides, free fatty acids has been demonstrated in cerebral venous thrombosis patients particularly when it complicates puerperium [9,17]. It has not been related to diet, although in the Indian subcontinent pregnant women are mostly fed with a high lipid diet in the ante- and post-natal periods.

The association of CVT with head injury, intracranial surgery, neoplasm, and arterio-venous malformation is most likely related to alteration in the blood coagulation and its decreased intravascular mobility.

Abnormalities in coagulation factor VII, deficiency of the heparin co-factor and anti-thrombin III have also been demonstrated in patients prone to cerebral venous thrombosis [21,22]. However, Bousser et al. [7] did not find any abnormalities in coagulation parameters as compared to normal controls. Anaemia has a significant role to play in the causation of CVT, more so in infants and children. The exact mechanism of this association is not known but it may be due to capillary ischaemia.

It is difficult to pinpoint the reasons for the increased incidence of sinus venous thrombosis in pregnancy and puerperium from the Indian subcontinent. Our own autopsy material of 39 cases of 'primary or aseptic' CVT include 25 cases in which puerperium was complicated with sinovenous occlusions [11]. The thrombus did not suggest infection. No source of infection in the body including the pelvic region was discernable. Retrograde embolisation from the pelvic venous plexus or intracranial vascular damage during labour as a cause of CVT does not explain its occurrence in the antepartum period. Moreover these factors fail to explain the occurrence of CVT as late as the 10th postpartum day.

There is still no clear-cut documentation of hypercoagulable state during pregnancy and puerperium. The various studies on blood coagulation factors and lipid contents are still to reveal the hypercoagulation in all the cases unequivocally. It is on these grounds that the cause of CVT during puerperium has been labelled 'primary'. The mechanism of CVT with the use of oral contraceptive steroids is explainable on the basis of an increase in the level of prothrombin, blood clotting factors such as VII, IX and X, plasminogen and antifibrinolytic activity within a few days to months after starting the oral pills.

Other factors

Haemodynamic factors may be important in congestive heart failure and dehydration. In some of the male patients cortical vein and sinus thrombus was related to the toxic effects of illicit alcohol [10]. Its association with Behcet's disease may be acceptable. The underlying mechanism however remains obscure. The pathogenesis by and large remains unknown where CVT is associated with cerebral vascular malformation, arachnoid cyst, brain neoplasm, diabetes mellitus, nephrotic syndrome, ulcerative colitis, and herpes zoster ophthalmaticus. It may be presumed that the underlying cause in these cases is vasculitis. Similarly anaemia, malnutrition, and cachexia have been reported in a number of patients with CVT although the exact nature of the lesion caused by these factors is unknown. It is also unclear why the deep cerebral sinuses are more often involved in infants and children.

Pathology

Topographically the lesions follow distinct patterns according to the veins and sinuses involved. Involvement of the temporal lobe by occlusion of the veins of Labbe and the lateral sinuses is rare (Fig. 1). The occlusion of a dural venous sinus alone may not cause significant alteration in the brain [24]. Brain infarction develops on extension of thrombosis to superficial cerebral veins, the Galenic venous system and the straight sinus. The brain is swollen, oedematous and heavy with a mottled grey cyanotic discolouration of the external surface. The overlying meninges are invariably blood-stained and contain cord-like rigid occluded veins. Narrowing of the ventricles and shifts across the midline are proportionate to the extent of infarction and its duration. Superior sagittal sinus examination shows a thrombus with alternate red and grey zones completely occluding the lumen. More advanced cases show a haemorrhagic infarction of the brain (Fig. 2). Microscopically there is variable degree of neuronal loss and damage. Affected neurones are shrunken and deeply stained. Leucocyte and macrophage reaction is slight and haemosiderin reaction is not evident. The type of cellular reaction does not age the venous infarct which is otherwise an important parameter in infarct of arterial origin.

Longer survival provides an opportunity to observe late changes such as

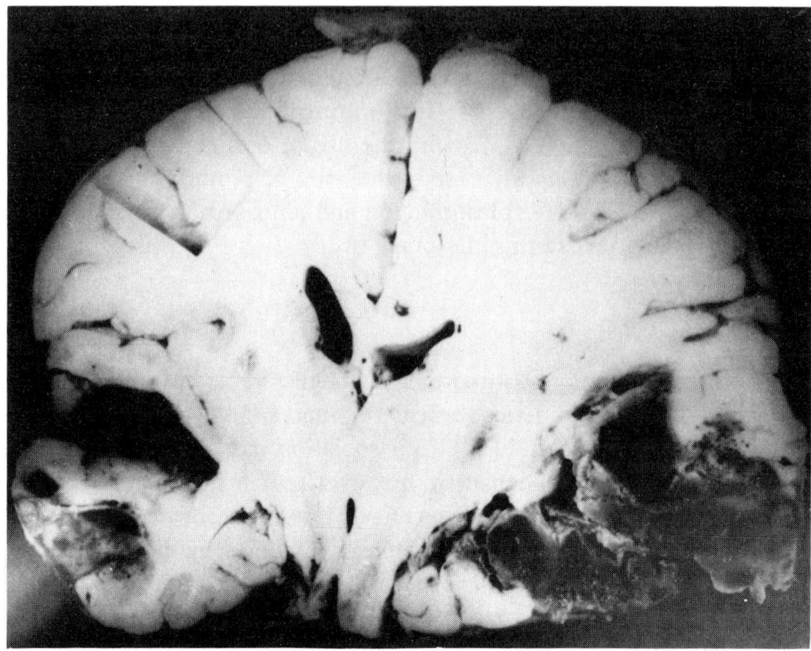

Fig. 1. Twenty five year-old female with diffuse headache, generalised seizures, aphasia and altered sensorium eleven days after delivery of a stillborn foetus. The autopsy six days later revealed thrombosis of the left transverse sinus, both the veins of Labbe and several other superficial cerebral veins. The left temporal lobe was swollen and showed uncal herniation. Cut section demonstrated bilateral temporal lobe haemorrhagic infarction.

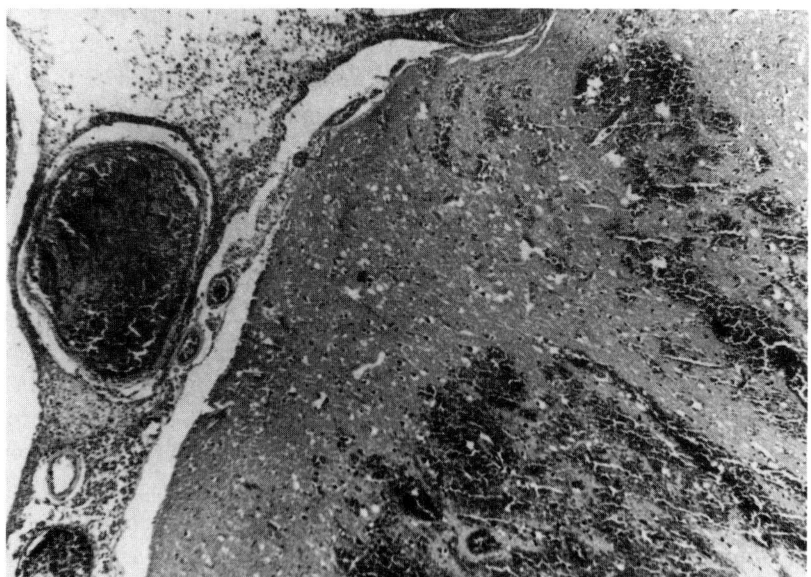

Fig. 2. Twenty two year-old female who died 17 days after a full term, normal delivery. Confluent haemorrhagic necrosis is associated with massive oedema in the left frontal lobe. Cut section of the occluded superior longitudinal sinus is seen in the sagittal plane.

organised thrombus, focal cortical atrophy and hydrocephalus. In infants and children liquefaction and cavitation of the white matter is frequently seen [24]. The superficial cerebral veins may show organised thrombus.

Diagnosis

A high degree of suspicion in infants and children and in the setting of puerperium, hypercoagulable states with symptoms such as headache, motor weakness and convulsions should raise suspicion of CVT. Appropriate investigations should rule out cerebral arterial occlusions, toxaemia of pregnancy, seizures complicating pregnancy, meningitis, benign raised intracranial tension, encephalopathies and intracranial tumours. In arterial occlusions seizures are rare, hemiparesis is dense, papilloedema is absent, CSF is normal and morbidity is more common than mortality. Positive angiographic findings are also more common.

Low haemoglobin levels, an increase in sedimentation rate and leukocytosis more than 10,000/cmm have been reported in 50 to 60% of cases. Focal or diffuse slowing in EEG with an epileptiform focus is seen in about 20% of cases [7,25]. Cerebrospinal fluid may reveal 10–200 cells/cmm with mild to moderate increase in protein. Occasionally CSF may be heavily blood-stained. We have performed lumbar CSF in 31 out of 55 cases of puerperal CVT [14]. In most cases a minimal increase in protein content and/or RBC up to 10 per high field was seen. Xanthochromia and frank haemorrhage was observed in only two cases each.

Radiology

Various radiological investigations that can delineate intracranial venous occlusion accurately and precisely are: angiography, computed tomography (CT) and magnetic resonance imaging (MRI).

Angiography

Carotid angiography continues to be an important investigation which can confirm the diagnosis with certainty. An increase in the arteriovenous circulation time is a constant feature in acute and subacute occlusions of the dural veins and sinuses. Delayed films taken at an interval of 5 to 12 sec help better visualisation of venous phase, more so in raised intracranial pressure. Non-filling of occluded sinus and or draining cerebral veins of the area corresponding to the neurological deficit is possibly the most definite objective finding suggestive of CVT. There may be abnormally dilated draining vessels, cork screw vessels which do not reach cortical surfaces, reversal of normal venous flow or vessel displacement caused by haemorrhagic infarct. The diagnostic yield can be improved by venous substraction angiography, selective carotid injections, and digital substraction angiography.

Computed tomography

CT scan is a useful investigation although the appearances are variable and nonspecific. The 'cord'-like hyperdensity is caused by clotted blood in the sinus, which looks like a triangle in the axial and on coronal sections. The centre of the triangle becomes less dense as haemoglobin within the clot is slowly removed. This results in 'empty delta sign' and is highly suggestive of intracranial sino-venous thrombosis . This sign becomes evident within 3–4 days after the onset of illness [26] (Fig. 3).

The cerebral oedema causes small ventricles. Infarct (haemorrhagic or non-haemorrhagic) leads to tentorial and/or gyral enhancements. The latter has been attributed to increase in blood flow across the collaterals and stasis of blood or hyperaemia [13]. The CT may be normal when a thrombotic process affects the cerebral veins more than the dural sinuses. CT is a less sensitive procedure for the diagnosis of cavernous sinus thrombosis. However, asymmetry in shape of lateral walls of cavernous sinus with abnormal low attenuated areas within the sinus is suggestive of sinus thrombosis (Fig. 4).

Magnetic resonance imaging

Macchi et al. [27] described magnetic resonance imaging (MRI) findings specific to sino-venous thrombosis in three female patients. In the initial phase of occlusion the normally occurring flow void is not seen in any plane. Venous collaterals confirm the haemodynamic alterations that have occurred secondarily to sino-venous thrombosis.

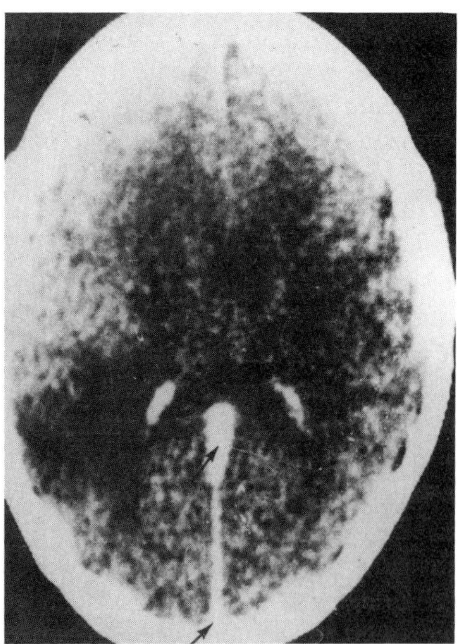

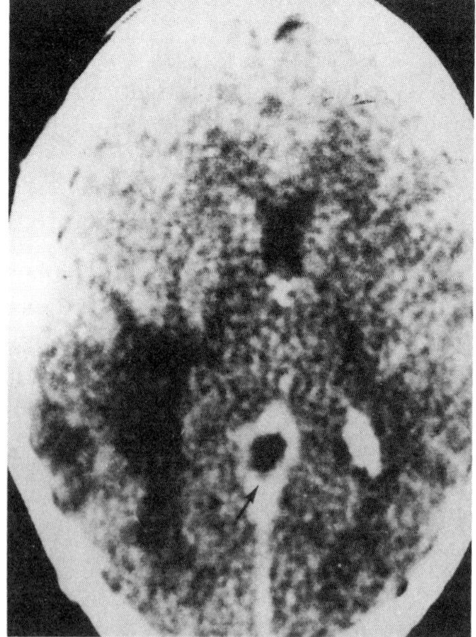

Fig. 3. Cord sign (arrows in a) and empty Delta sign (arrow in b) in the CT scan of a young female in whom puerperium was complicated with CVT. CT findings in the patient show involvement of the vein of Galen, straight sinus and superior sagittal sinus.

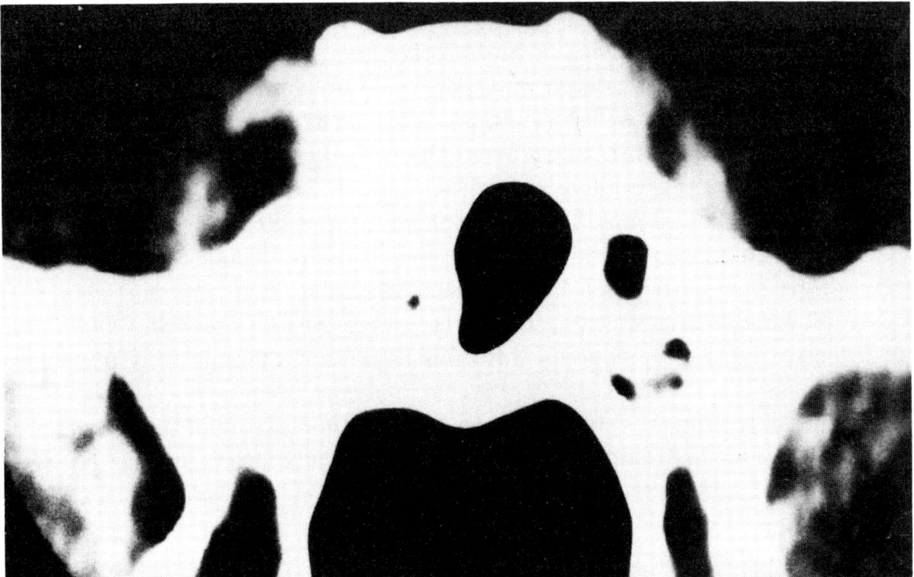

Fig. 4. Twenty five year-old female who suffered bilateral cavernous sinus thrombosis following tubal recanalisation surgery. CT scan shows convexity of lateral walls of the sinus (arrows) with an irregular hypodens area in it suggestive of an organising thrombus.

These are seen on T1 weighted images in which vessel appears isodense. On T2 weighted images the thrombus appears hypodense due to deoxyhaemoglobin in the intact red blood cells. Flow void reappears later, once the recanalisation of the vessel sets in. It seems that MRI will replace the utility of angiography and CT in confirming the clinical diagnosis of intracranial sinus venous thrombosis.

Treatment

Seizures and raised intracranial pressure may be life threatening and require immediate attention. Measures to prevent the extension of thrombosis into normal vessels need to be taken. Antibiotics should be administered in septic cases and hypertension controlled to minimize the risk of intracranial bleeding. Neurogenic hypertension from Cushing's effect should not be tampered with since it can lead to decrease in cerebral blood flow in the setting of raised intracranial pressure. Treatment is primarily medical. Routine measures for the care of comatosed patients are self-evident. Ideally the patient should be treated in an intensive care unit.

Seizures are relatively resistant to treatment, are common and status epilepticus is frequent. Intravenous diazepam infusion up to a maximum of 70 mg in 24 h is recommended. Diphenylhydantoin sodium is given in the usual dosage. The prophylactic usage of anticonvulsants and its duration remains controversial. Some have recommended prophylactic anticonvulsants if EEG shows seizure activity.

We recommend anticonvulsants for 3–5 years provided there are no seizures during this period and the EEG is not grossly abnormal.

Cerebral oedema is life-threatening. Cytotoxic oedema of early stage is soon followed by vasogenic oedema within 24 to 48 h. Parenteral dexamethasone efficacy in this condition is not proven. Other medical measures to check raised intracranial pressure are fluid restriction, use of frusemide and hyperosmotic agents. However, there may be risk of dehydration resulting from such measures which can promote the thrombotic process [8]. Low molecular weight dextran to improve the microcirculation is advocated especially in infants and children in whom dehydration is suspected. Recurrent lumbar puncture provides a temporary but effective means of reducing intracranial pressure, though it is not without risk.

The aim of treating the thrombosis is to prevent progression of the thrombus and promote early recanalisation. The fibrinolytic activator urokinase has been used successfully [25,28]. Frequent monitoring with CT is recommended in view of potential dangers of this drug to initiate secondary intracranial haemorrhage. The use of this drug has also been shown to be detrimental [29]. Opinions on the use of anticoagulants are sharply divided. The venous infarction is mostly haemorrhagic and use of anticoagulants can promote intracranial bleeding. Objective data on which to base any decision are not available. A non-haemorrhagic infarct may become haemorrhagic in its natural course and an early substitution of anticoagulant therapy in this situation may do harm. In our opinion serial CT scan studies are a useful parameter in determining the use of anticoagulants. Extension of the cerebral lesion requires its use whereas if it becomes haemorrhagic one may have to stop the anticoagulants.

Heparin is used intramuscularly or intravenously in different dosage schedule; 5000 IU 4 hourly to 15,000 IU 8 hourly. The anticoagulants should be continued for a minimum period of 2–3 weeks to cover postpartum hypercoagulable state. Heparin should be used for 6 weeks followed by oral anticoagulants for a period of 6 months when CVT is associated with deep leg vein thrombosis. Salicylic acid is known to decrease platelet adhesiveness, which was found to be increased in patients of CVT. Its beneficial use is not established clearly.

Surgery is performed to decompress the brain under tension. Evacuation of localised haemorrhage at times hampers with the beneficial plugging effect of the clot and thus can result in secondary haemorrhage. Most of the patients on whom decompression by way of craniotomy and temporal lobectomy was performed were moribund and had haemorrhagic infarct. Nagpal [10] performed surgery on 34 out of 80 cases. The large mass effect in all these cases was produced by haemorrhagic infarction. Fourteen of these patients died following surgery, 18 improved and 2 remained unchanged. These patients had high mortality compared to those treated conservatively.

Prognosis

It is difficult to form an opinion of the outcome of this disorder. Prognostic gloom in surgically treated patients is probably false as most of these patients were very sick at the time of surgical intervention.

The mortality of puerperal CVT ranges from 26 to 37%. Undoubtedly the outlook is worse in infancy. Ebbs' (1937) gloomy picture of the outcome in children is true even today. It is because of its rapidity of onset, early spread of thrombosis to the deep venous system, delayed onset of symptoms caused by elastic skull and the tendency of unmyelinated white matter of the infant brain to liquify.

It has been observed that recovery is rapid and complete if the patient survives the acute episode. The functional recovery of cases who survive is quick, reasonably good and is better than in arterial stroke. The majority who survive have no significant disability. Recovery starts within weeks or months, although it is not possible to predict the course of a given case.

Alteration in sensorium, poorly controlled seizures, status epilepticus, tachycardia and respiratory disturbances, association of deep vein thrombosis elsewhere and involvement of deep intracranial venous system carry bad prognosis. Mental retardation, cortico spinal motor weakness such as spastic diplegia may be observed in infants who survive. Epilepsy is a troublesome and common long term complication. Red blood cells in CSF, paralytic signs and even altered sensorium may not always predict a bad prognosis. From our experience many of such patients improved significantly.

Acknowledgements

We are grateful to Dr A.R. Banerjee, Prof. of Morbid Anatomy, Postgraduate Institute of Medical Education and Research, Chandigarh, India for his contributions to Figs. 1 and 2 in this article.

References

1. Averback P (1978) Primary cerebral venous thrombosis in young adults, the diverse manifestations of an under recognised disease. Ann. Neurol. 3: 81–86.
2. Banerjee AK (1974) Cerebral venous thrombosis in men. Bull. PGI, Chandigarh, India, 8: 88–91.
3. Kalbag RM and Woolf AL (1967) Cerebral venous thrombosis. Oxford University Press, London.
4. Caroll JD, Leak D and Lee HA (1966) Cerebral thrombophlebitis in pregnancy and the puerperium. Quart. J. Med. 35: 347–368.
5. Srinivasan K (1983) Cerebral venous and arterial thrombosis in pregnancy and puerperium: A study of 135 patients. Angiology 34: 731–746.
6. Krayenbuhl HA (1967) Cerebral venous and sinus thrombosis. Clin. Neurosurg. 14: 1–24.
7. Bousser MG, Chiras J, Bories J and Castaigne P (1985) Cerebral venous thrombosis – A review of 38 cases. Stroke 16: 199–213.

8. Gates PC and Barnett HJM (1986) In: Barnett HJM, Stein BM, Mohr JP and Yatsu FM (eds.) Cortical veins stroke pathophysiology, diagnosis and management. Churchill Livingstone, New York, pp. 731–746.
9. Bansal BC, Gupta RR and Prakash C (1980) Stroke during pregnancy and puerperium in young females below the age of 40 years as a result of cerebral venous/venous sinus thrombosis. Jpn. Heart J. 21: 171–183.
10. Nagpal RD (1983) Dural sinus and cerebral venous thrombosis. Neurosurg. Rev. 6: 155–160.
11. Chopra JS and Banerjee AK (1989) In: Vinken PJ, Bruyn GW and Toole J (eds.) Primary intracranial sinovenous occlusions in pregnancy, puerperium, neonates and juveniles. Handbook of Clinical Neurology. New Series, Strokes vol. 2, Elsevier, Amsterdam.
12. Cottrill CM and Kaplan S (1973) Cerebral vascular accidents in cyanotic congenital heart disease. Am. J. Dis. Child 125: 484–487.
13. Chiras J, Bousser MG, Meder JF, Koussa A and Bories J (1985) CT in cerebral thrombophlebitis. Neuroradiology 27: 145–154.
14. Bansal SR and Chopra JS (1988) Cortical venous thrombosis a retrospective study of eighty three cases. Paper read at 38th annual conference of NSI, Chandigarh, India, December.
15. Srinivasan K and Natarajan M (1974) Cerebral venous and arterial thrombosis in pregnancy and puerperim: A study of 90 patients. Neurol. Ind. 22: 131–140.
16. Solomon GE, Engel M, Hecht HL and Rapoport AR (1982) Progressive dyskinesia due to internal cerebral vein thrombosis. Neurology 32: 769–772.
17. Chopra JS, Prabhakar SK, Das KC, Chakravarthy RN, Sodhi JS and Wahi PL (1979) In: Greenhalgh M and Rose FC (eds.) Stroke in the young in North-West India. Progress in stroke research (1st Ed.) Pitman Medical, Bath, England, pp. 217–235.
18. Girolami A, Pardatscher K, Scanarini M, Job I and Patrass G (1980) Clotting changes in two patients with longitudinal sinus thrombosis. Haemostasis 9: 71–78.
19. Bonnar J, McNicol GP and Douglas AJ (1969) Fibrinolytic enzyme system and pregnancy. Br. Med. J. 3: 387–388.
20. Chopra JS and Prabhakar 8 (1979) Clinical features and risk factors in stroke in young. Acta Neurol. Scand. 60: 289–300.
21. Kobayashi S, Hino H and Tazaki Y (1980) Superior sagittal sinus thrombosis due to familial anithrombin III deficiency: A case report of two families. Rinsho Shinkeisakis 20: 904–910.
22. Komiyami A, Kawamura M, Kirayama K, Kitano K and Oh H (1985) Cerebral venous thrombosis with familial antithrombin III deficiency. No-To-Shinkei 37: 589–594.
23. Chopra JS, Prabhakar S and Chakravarty RN (1980) A prospective study of lipid and coagulation parameters in stroke in young. Ind. J. Med. Res. 72: 731–738.
24. Kalbag PM and Woolf AL (1972) In: Vinken PJ and Bruyn GW (eds.) Thrombosis and thrombophlebitis of the cerebral veins and dural sinus. Handbook of Clinical Neurology. vol. 12, Elsevier, Amsterdam, pp. 422–446.
25. Vines FS and Davis DO (1971) Clinical-radiological correlation in cerebral venous occlusive disease. Radiology 98: 9–22.
26. Buonanno FS, Moody DM, Ball MR and Laster DW (1978) Computed cranial tomographic findings in cerebral sinovenous occlusion. J. Comp. Assis. Tomography 2: 281–290.
27. Macchi PJ, Grossman RT, Gommri JM, Goldberg HI, Zimmerman RA and Bilaniuk LT (1986) High field MR imaging of cerebral venous thrombosis. J. Comp. Assis. Tomography 10: 10–15.
28. Rocco CD, Lannelli A, Leone M and Valori VM (1981) Heparin urokinase treatment in aseptic dural sinus thrombosis. Arch. Neurol. 38: 431–435.
29. Gattelfinger DM and Kokmen E (1977) Superior sagittal sinus thrombosis. Arch. Neurol. 34: 2–6.

Transient ischemic attacks (TIA)

James F. Toole and Walter C. Teagle
Stroke Research Center, Wake Forest University, Winston-Salem, NC 27103, USA

Dr Ernesto Herskovits, Vice-President of the World Federation of Neurology for Latin America and a very active contributor to the Research Group on Cerebrovascular Disorders, died unexpectedly and prematurely on the 4th of March 1988. He was to present this portion of our program and I am proud to substitute for him and to deliver this presentation in his memory.

Professor Herskovits was deeply committed to the advancement of neurology not only in his own country but throughout Latin America and the world, and we all mourn his loss.

Transient ischemic attack (TIA) is the rubric used to classify patients with episodes of focal neurologic deficit of sudden onset, which resolve completely in less than 24 h, and which leaves no residual damage to the nervous system. By common agreement this includes transient monocular blindness (amaurosis fugax) but excludes syncope, vertigo, migraine and convulsions. Episodes that last longer than 24 h but fully resolve within a week or two are called reversible ischemic neurologic deficit (RIND) and are thought to be transitional between TIA and infarction in which the deficit can persist permanently. However, these definitions were developed before the advent of cranial computed tomography, magnetic resonance imaging and positron emission tomography, all of which have demonstrated long lasting and sometimes even permanent damage in patients whose event resolved completely within the 24 h time frame which has been accepted clinically as the upper time limit for TIA [15].

The gravity of what TIA signifies is underscored by the fact that in the Caucasian population of the United States, the likelihood of stroke occurring in persons 65 to 74 years of age is about 1% per year, but in a matched TIA population the probability increases from 5 to 8% per year [17,23].

The Mayo Clinic community survey recorded preceding TIA in almost 50% of patients with atherothrombotic infarction, in 20 to 25% of lacunar infarctions and in approximately 10% of all cerebral emboli [20]. Others have reported similar or somewhat different findings [17,18,23–25].

TIAs are more common in whites than in blacks or orientals, probably because of the greater prevalence of atherosclerosis in the white population [19,21,22,26]. Men are affected twice as frequently as women, and the onset occurs most often in the 50 to 70 year age group. About 90% of TIAs occur in the carotid distribution, 7% in the vertebral-basilar, and 3% in both [11,12].

More than 7% of those who have a TIA suffer stroke within the year and is followed by stroke in perhaps 30% within 5 years. A TIA patient has about a 5 times greater risk of suffering a stroke than a patient of same age without TIA. Furthermore, the first month after a TIA is the most dangerous so that a TIA is an indicator for urgent evaluation and initiation of therapy [2,6,13].

Pathogenesis

In the 1960–1970s, it was believed that the cause of TIAs was episodic hypotension [28,30,32], cardiac dysrhythmia, or low perfusion distal to tight stenosis [14]. Now ultrasound and angiography frequently demonstrate ulcerated plaques in the extracranial portions of the internal carotid artery and hypotension is seldom found [31]. It was, however, the landmark publication by Dalal (1965) which crystallised the belief that most TIAs are embolic in nature. He depicted evanescent embolic obstructions within leptomeningeal arteries. It is suspected that many more emboli traverse the brain's vascular bed than are recognised by patients, and that the process is much more dynamic than has previously been suspected, so that the episodes we recognise are only a fraction of the real number of emboli which impact upon the cerebral circulation.

Although TIAs have many causes, atherosclerosis is the most common. Aggregations of fibrin, platelets, or cholesterol crystals have been seen in the optic fundus during and soon after TIAs and so it is assumed that similar microemboli are responsible for the cerebral episodes.

There is suspicion that the pathogenetic mechanism of TIAs persisting for less than 60 min differs from those of longer duration. Those shorter than 30 min are probably due to artery-to-artery microemboli, whereas the ones of longer duration have a greater probability of being a larger size and from the valves or chambers of the left heart.

Although there are as many varieties of TIA as there are brain functions, episodes are often stereotyped in the same individual. The patient suddenly becomes aware that a portion of his normal neural function process is lost. Most commonly, there is a loss of power. Other patients with sensory involvement describe numbness or peculiar sensation not akin to any previously experienced, although some compare it to the lack of feeling that follows a nerve block for dental anesthesia. It is specifically not painful or tingling.

Episodic behavioural abnormality or amnesia may be a manifestation of TIA if the limbic system is involved. Limb shaking, consisting of brief involuntary coarse movement of arm or leg, can be an unusual manifestation of TIA.

Some attacks are characterised by partial or complete blindness of one or both eyes. This dramatic event, which one imagines would frighten the patient, generally subsides too rapidly for panic to ensue but it is usually sufficient to make the patient seek medical attention quickly. The type of symptoms enhance or decrease the probability that the patient will seek medical attention.

Almost invariably TIAs develop from their first manifestation to full expression within a minute. This extraordinary rapidity is a hallmark, subjective though it is, which is very useful for differentiating TIA from migraine or focal sensory or motor convulsion. This brevity is one of the major arguments for the pathogenesis of most TIAs being embolic in nature.

Almost half of TIAs persist for less than 5 min, another quarter subside within an hour, and the remainder are gone within 24 h. Those lasting less than 1 h are more likely to be caused by a microembolism from an artery, whereas those persisting longer tend to originate from the heart. Generally speaking, the time taken from the moment the attack is first noted until its height is less than the time taken for recovery to occur after symptoms begin to diminish.

It is a good general rule that episodes which last longer than 24 h signify infarction or some other pathologic process; but there are occasional cases which take days for complete resolution. Although the pathogenetic mechanism of these prolonged attacks may be the same as those of short duration, they are classified as infarction with recovery or as a reversible ischemic neurologic deficit (RIND).

Frequency

Some patients suffer only one episode in a lifetime and others as many as 12 to 20 very brief attacks in one day. Closely approximated episodes and especially their increasing frequency is an ominous sign which often portends infarction. Therefore, these crescendo TIAs are an alerting mechanism for speedy evaluation and appropriate management of the patient. In most cases, however, there are fewer than one or two attacks per week and occasionally less than one a month.

When the history and clinical findings suggest a vascular disorder, the physician must determine its pathogenesis and triggering mechanisms before concluding that the patient is suffering from atherothrombotic disease. Even if atherosclerosis is the probable cause, the physician must still ascertain what precipitated the attack and whether some other unrelated disease contributed to its symptoms.

There is increasing realisation that the atheroma itself is often not the culprit of the TIAs or cerebral infarction. Rather, it is the ulceration which can occur in plaque. These ulcers may cause clinical phenomena due to platelet emboli or other embolic materials. Blood clots within ulcers often propagate, resulting in an indentation with a tail extending into the bloodstream.

Course and Prognosis

Of TIA patients who eventually develop infarction, the short time often elapsing between the two determines that these patients be evaluated urgently and treated as emergencies. About 36% have infarction within a month and 50% within 12 months of onset of TIAs.

Five-year mortality rates in TIA patients average about 20 to 25%. However, the majority of these fatalities are secondary to myocardial rather than cerebral infarction.

In our Wake Forest experience [1,2], we found a great variation in the five year survival of our selected cohort of TIA patients, from over 95% for a 60 year-old without excess risk, to less than 25% for all those with excess risk. Although the survival of strata differed, the average mortality was about one-half that found in our previous analysis of similar cohort during 1961–1973, demonstrating within our own patient experience the remarkable decline in stroke mortality that has occurred during the past 25 years.

To a large degree, prognosis of TIA depends upon its aetiology and concomitant diseases. Younger populations in which excess risk is generally less, aetiologies such as valvular heart and congenital heart disease, and hypotension are major contributors to TIA. In the elderly, hypertension and atherosclerosis become major contributors to risk in the course and prognosis is poorest.

The indiscriminate use of aspirin has altered the prognosis so that all the data accumulated before 1975 which contribute to the natural history of untreated TIA can no longer be utilised.

The platelet anti-aggregator, ASA, helps prevent stroke and myocardial infarction [3–5]. Combinations with dipyridamole might perhaps foster effectiveness. However, the dose of both drugs for optimal antithrombotic efficacy is still unresolved.

There is no doubt that haemorheological and haemostasiological factors are involved in active cerebral ischaemia and do adversely reflect on the nutritional, metabolic and functional capacity of brain tissue by hampering cerebral microcirculation. The haemorrheological properties can be improved by medication such as ticlopidine or pentoxifylline, which improves cerebral capillary perfusion [8,11,17,23].

Dr Herskovits and his group were investigating the comparative effects of pentoxifylline and ASA at the time of his death [29]. They concluded that both treatments resulted in fewer recurrent ischemic episodes that would be expected without treatment. Lower rate of recurrence of ischemic events was found in patients treated with pentoxifylline (14%) compared to 24.1% in the ASA group. The overall results of treatment show statistically slight superiority in favour of pentoxifylline ($P = 0.087$). Thus, pentoxifylline when given in three divided doses of 400 mg in slow release formulation may therefore be a useful agent for reducing risk of TIA and infarction [7,9].

Whether in the long run medical, surgical, or a combination of both based upon individual case selection will eventually prove to be the therapy of choice awaits further data from current on-going studies.

References

1. Howard G, Toole JF, Frye-Pierson J and Hinshelwood LC (1987) Factors influencing the survival of 451 transient ischemic attack patients. Stroke 18: 552–557.
2. Howard G, Brockschmidt JK, Rose LA, Frye-Pierson JL, Crouse JR, Evans GW, Mitchell ES and Toole JF (1989) Changes in survival after transient ischemic attacks: Observations comparing the 1970s and 1980s. Neurology 39: 9822–9985.
3. Canadian Cooperative Study Group (1978) A randomized trial of aspirin and sulfinpyrazone in threatened stroke. N. Engl. J. Med. 299: 53–59.
4. Fields WS, Lemak HA, Frankowski RF et al. (1980) Controlled trial of aspirin in cerebral ischaemia. Circulation 62 (Suppl. V): 90–96.
5. Millikan CH and McDowell FH (1978) Treatment of transient ischemic attacks. Stroke 9: 299–308.
6. Warlow C (1985) Transient ischemic attacks: Current treatment concepts. Drugs 29: 474–482.
7. Hartmann A (1985) Comparative randomized study of cerebral blood flow after long-term administration of Pentoxifylline and co-dergocrine-mesylate in patients with chronic cerebrovascular disease. Curr. Med. Res. Opin. 9: 475–479.
8. Ott E and Lechner H (1983) Changes of flow properties of blood in cerebrovascular disease and their medical treatment with pentoxifylline. J. Cereb. Blood Flow Metabol. 3(1): 530–531.
9. Toole JF, Yuson CP, Janeway R, Johnston F, Davis C, Cordell AR and Howard G (1978) Transient ischemic attacks: A prospective study of 225 patients. Neurology 28: 746–753.
10. Fisher CM (1962) Concerning recurrent transient cerebral ischemic attacks. Can. Med. Assoc. J. 86: 1091–1099.
11. Johnson SE and Harvard S (1986) Transient cerebral ischemic attacks in the young and middle aged. A population study. Stroke 4: 662.
12. Millikan CH (1965) The pathogenesis of transient focal cerebral ischaemia. The Lewis A. Connor Memorial Lecture. Circulation 32: 438–445.
13. Caplan LR (1981) Are terms such as completed stroke or RIND of continued usefulness? Stroke 14: 431.
14. Boysen G, Jensen G and Schnohr P (1978) Focal cerebral transient ischemic attacks: A population study from Copenhagen. Acta Neurol. Scand. 58 (suppl. 67): 221.
15. Wang CC, Cheng XM, Li SZ, Bolis CL and Schoenberg BS (1983) Epidemiology of cerebrovascular disease in an urban community of Beijing, People's Republic of China. Neuroepidemiology 2: 121.
16. Li SC, Schoenberg BS, Wang CC, Cheng XM, Bolis CL and Wang KJ (1985) Cerebrovascular disease in the People's Republic of China: Epidemiologic and clinical features. Neurology 35: 1708.
17. Whisnant JP (1976) A population study of stroke and TIA, Rochester, Minnesota. In: Gillingham FJ, Mawdsley C and Williams AE (eds.) Stroke. Churchill Livingstone, Edinburgh, p. 5.
18. Ueda K, Kiyohara Y, Hasuo Y, Yanai T, Kawano H, Wada J, Kato I, Kajiwara E, Omae T and Fujishima M (1987) Transient cerebral ischemic attacks in a Japanese community, Hisayama, Japan. Stroke 18: 844.
19. Friedman GD, Wilson WS, Moner JM, Colandrea MA and Nichaman MA (1969) Transient ischemic attacks in a community. J.A.M.A. 210: 1428.
20. Rhoads GG, Popper JS, Kagan A and Yano K (1980) Incidence of transient ischemic cerebral ischemic attack in Hawaiian Japanese men: The Honolulu heart study. Stroke 11: 21.
21. Zupping R and Roose M (1976) Epidemiology of cerebrovascular disease in Tartu, Estonia, USSR, 1970–1973. Stroke 7: 187.
22. Mettinger KL, Soderstrom CE and Allender E (1984) Epidemiology of acute cerebrovascular disease before the age of 55 in the Stockholm county, 1973–1977. I. Incidence and mortality rates. Stroke 15: 795.
23. Terent A (1979) A prospective epidemiological survey of cerebrovascular disease in a Swedish community. Uppsala J. Med. Sci. 84: 235.
24. Alter M, Sobel E, McCoy RL, Francis ME, Shoger F, Lewitt LP and Meehan EF (1985) Stroke in the Lehigh Valley, incidence based on a community-wide hospital register. Neuroepidemiology 4: 1.

25. Heistad DD, Williams JK, Baumbach GL, Faraci FM and Armstrong ML (1989) Hypothesis: Vasospasm contributes to amaurosis and transient cerebral ischaemia. J. Cereb. Blood Flow Metab. 9 (suppl. 1).
26. Gurdjian ES and Thomas LM (1969) Cerebral vasospasm. Surg. Gynecol. Obstet. 129: 931–948.
27. Bogousslavsky J and Regli F (1983) Delayed TIAs distal to bilateral occlusion of carotid arteries: Evidence for embolic and haemodynamic mechanisms. Stroke 14: 58–61.
28. Fazekas JF and Alman RW (1964) The role of hypotension in transitory focal cerebral ischaemia. Am. J. Med. Sci. 248: 567–570.
29. Herskovits E, Famulari A, Tamaroff L, Gonzalez AM, Vazques A, Dominguez R, Fraiman H, Vila J, Benjamin V and Matera V (1989) Comparative study of pentoxifylline vs anti-aggregants in patients with transient ischemic attacks. Acta Neurol. Scand. (suppl.) 127: 31–35.

Strokes (CVD) in the young

Praful M. Dalal et al.
Sir H.N. Hospital Medical Research Society, R.R. Roy Road, Bombay 400 004, India

Introduction

Cerebrovascular Disease (CVD) or stroke is one of the foremost causes of high morbidity and mortality for many nations of the world, posing a major socio-economic challenge in occupational neuro-rehabilitational programmes of 'stroke-survivors'. For example, in the USA alone it has been estimated that a sum of 3261 million dollars is spent as direct cost for treatment, in addition to 4104 million dollars as indirect costs consequent on economic losses of 'stroke victims' [1].

Review of literature

Magnitude of problem

Community based surveys from USA, Europe and Japan indicate average annual incidence rates of 111 to 180 per 100,000 population, and 9 to 28 per 100,000 young persons (under 45 years). Similarly, the approximate point prevalence rate has ranged from 400 to 700 per 100,000 population and 150 to 200 per 100,000 for the young [2–4] (Table 1). The available information on stroke mortality is summarised in Table 2.

For the Indian subcontinent, epidemiological information on annual incidence or prevalence rates and morbidity and mortality trends in defined populations are not available. The point prevalence rate in semiurban areas of Vellore for 'hemiplegia' (? CVD) has been reported at 56.9 per 100,000 persons [5], but there are numerous difficulties in validation of stroke diagnosis in population surveys [6]. Likewise, Hatano [7] has critically analysed similar difficulties in accuracy of stroke diagnosis and 'observer variations' in the multicentric W.H.O. Stroke Study. Nonetheless, available information on mortality trends for Asian-Pacific countries has been compiled in Table 2 [8–10]. Here, *it is important to note that the age distribution population structure of Asian people having a life expectancy of about 58 years, and where 50% of our people are under the age of 20, is remarkably different and not at all comparable to Japanese, European and American populations.* The approximate annual age specific incidence rate for strokes in young

Table 1. Distribution of strokes in young (< 45 years) subjects (male and female) and annual incidence rates per 100,000 population (1971–1974)[a]

Study area	Total population	Total CVD cases (N)	No. of young cases (n)	Annual incidence rates	% of young cases
Europe					
Gothenburg	450,900	784	92	8	(11.73)
Frederiksberg	100,000	891	13	7	(1.46)
Dublin	133,700	539	29	9	(5.38)
Espoo	103,500	303	34	19	(11.22)
North Karelia	178,300	938	69	20	(7.36)
Zagreb	87,900	631	23	11	(3.65)
Middle East					
Zerifin	218,400	916	12	11[d]	(1.31)
Africa					
Ibadan[e]	803,100	300	93	4	(31.00)
Asia					
Akita	36,100	382	29	24	(7.59)
Saku	105,200	708	27	39[d]	(3.81)
Ulan Bator	261,300	653	59	6	(9.04)
Rohtak[c,e]	124,700	82	9	3	(10.98)
Colombo[c]	662,400	163	17	4	(10.43)
Vellore[b,e]	258,576	147	40	NA	(27.21)

[a]WHO collaborative study on the control of stroke in the community (1980); [b]Non-WHO study; [c]Joined the study later; [d]Annual incidence rate grouped < 45 to 54 yrs; [e]Age groups slightly different: < 40 years, 40–49 years, etc.; NA = Not available.

subjects (35–44 years) is remarkably low, in the range 9 (rural) to 28 (urban) per 100,000 people [4] (Table 1); whereas a high percentage of young CVD cases by hospital admissions in India (13.4 to 32%) may be related to sample bias [5,11–21]. Here, several risk factors have been described and debated in ischemic CVD (ICVD) in the young [22,23]. Though longitudinal prospective community surveys are advisable [24], such studies for developing nations are expensive and the cost prohibitive [25].

There appears to be a significant decline in the incidence of CVD mortality [2]; though the relative distribution of CVD lesions (ischemic and haemorrhagic) in hospital cases has not changed over the years. Dalal et al. [26] have made similar observations from two prospective hospital based stroke studies (1963–1968; 1978–1982) in west-central India. This higher percentage of 'stroke-survivors' with varying residual disability is now posing a major socioeconomic challenge in occupational rehabilitation of stroke victims.

Table 2. Cerebrovascular disease: Average annual age-adjusted mortality rates for various countries (Source WHO/NINCDS CVD survey report (1967–1973))

Country	Years	Mortality rate[a] (per 100,000 population)
1. Occidental studies:		
North America		
USA	1967–1973	79.0
Canada	1967–1973	68.1
South America		
Mexico	1967–1973	48.0
Uruguay	1967–1973	113.4
Chile	1967–1973	97.1
Europe		
England/Wales	1967–1973	97.9
Sweden	1967–1973	63.9
Finland	1967–1973	121.4
West Germany	1967–1973	110.9
Italy	1967–1973	99.0
Denmark	1967–1973	65.9
France	1967–1973	85.0
Eastern Europe		
Czechoslovakia	1967–1973	121.6
Poland	1967–1973	39.6
2. Oriental studies:		
Asian-Pacific countries		
Oceania		
Australia	1967–1973	110.9
New Zealand	1967–1972	100.0
Asia		
Japan	1967–1973	196.7
Philippines	1967–1973	35.8
Taiwan[b]	1971	69.7
Hong Kong[b]	1970	45.8
Singapore[b]	1970	50.2
Middle East		
Israel	1967–1973	111.8

[a]Age adjusted to 1950 US population (Fratiglioni et al., 1983); [b]Viryavejakul, 1982 (separately calculated).

Materials and Methods

The data presented are obtained from a recently concluded multicentric prospective case-control study on RFs in cerebral infarction (CI), initiated by the Indian Council of Medical Research (ICMR) in different regions of India. For this prospective study, a standardised pretested protocol was used for collecting baseline and follow-up data with well defined inclusion and exclusion criteria [27]. The data base from our centre comprises 186 stroke subjects (93 under 41 years and 93 sequential cases over the age of 40) who had a recent ischemic stroke (6 weeks or less), 105 non-stroke hospital controls and '561' healthy community volunteers. In the statistical analysis, a total of 30 categorical variables were used for univariate analysis, to judge the prognostic significance of such variables for CI. For logist multivariate interactive regression analysis, a set of 17 variables was used. Computational work was also done using stepwise procedure with sub-program of statistical package social sciences (SPSS) to include all potential discriminating variables for eligible cases and controls by age and sex (Table 3). Statistically valid information was available in 114 stroke subjects, 63 non-stroke hospital controls and 286 'healthy' community volunteers. The latter sample was used for case-control analysis.

Results

Table 3 shows the standardised canonical discriminant function coefficients (df) for stepwise variable selection with minimum value of F necessary for entry set at 1.000 and minimum tolerance level at 0.001 at each step. Hypertension, diabetes mellitus, tobacco use and haemoglobin (Hgb) concentration rather than level of cholesterol have stood out as important RFs in atherothrombotic cerebral infarction in the young [27–30].

Discussion

In a developing country like India, with a population of over 750 million people, to ascertain the true incidence, mortality and morbidity rate and to study the RFs in strokes is an extremely difficult task. Most of the data published are from retrospective analyses of subjects admitted to urban medical hospitals whereas the majority of our people live in towns or villages. There is also lack of standardised stroke terminology and baseline investigations. Furthermore, necropsy verification of death certificates is an additional problem. Despite these limitations, analyses of data as collected from major urban university hospitals suggest that nearly 2% of all hospital cases, 4.5% of medical and 20% of neurological admissions are from CVD, and the incidence of strokes in younger persons (below 40 years) is high (13 to 32%) when compared to similar data from the western hemisphere, excluding African and Latin American countries.

Different RFs have been attributed to 'strokes in the young' by various Indian authors. A disturbed equilibrium in coagulation and fibrinolysis has been suggested in the aetiopathology of nonembolic cerebral infarction in the young [29,32,33] in North India. Srinivasan [34] considers meningovascular syphilis as an important RF for hospital cases in Madurai in South India. The possibility of subacute CNS infection (e.g., tubercular), arteritis and autoimmune angiitis as RF [18,28] needs careful re-evaluation. Ischemic cerebrovascular complications of pregnancy and puerperium is commonly seen throughout India and most of the

Table 3. Prospective case-control study of ischemic strokes

Discriminant analysis of 'Risk Factors' (RF)[a]
(Data base: 186 (P) + 666 (HCCC) = Tn 852)
(EP 114 + EC 349 = ET 463)

1. High blood sugar df (0.53)[a]
2. High blood pressure df (0.48)[a]
3. Tobacco use df (0.41)[a]
4. Low Haemoglobin df (–0.34)[a]

(P < 0.05)

Males

Young (≤ 40 years) (EP 39 + EC 69 = ET 108)	Elderly (> 40 years) (EP 32 + EC 124 = ET 156)
1. *Low haemoglobin* df (–0.69)	1. High blood sugar df (0.61)
2. Tobacco use (smoking) df (0.47)	2. High blood pressure df (0.49)
3. High blood sugar df (0.41)	3. *Low haemoglobin* df (–0.34)
4. High-blood pressure df (0.24)	4. Tobacco use (smoking) df (0.27)
(P < 0.05)	(P < 0.05)

Females

Young (≤ 40 years) (EP 19 + EC 69 = ET 88)	Elderly (> 40 years) (EP 24 + EC 87 = ET 111)
1. High blood pressure df (0.90)	1. High blood sugar df (0.49)
2. High blood sugar df (0.43)	2. High blood pressure df (0.38)
3. *Low haemoglobin* df (–0.39)	3. *Low haemoglobin* df (–0.22)
(P < 0.05)	(P < 0.05)

[a]Standardized Canonical Discriminant Function Coefficients (df); P = patients; HCCC = Hospital controls and community controls; EP = Eligible patients; EC = Eligible controls; ET = Eligible total.

cases are from cerebral venous thrombosis [29,34,35] occurring during perinatal period. Similar findings are also reported in the West [36]. Obesity, hyperuricaemia etc. are relatively uncommon potential RFs in our subjects [29–31].

The recent ICMR prospective multicentric stroke study showed hypertension, elevated blood sugar, low concentration of normal Hgb and use of tobacco as important RFs. HBP was seen in both the sexes at all ages. Similar relationship between CVD and HBP has been reported in the Japanese [37] and American studies. In the literature, diabetes mellitus is listed as one of the RFs contributing to stroke morbidity and mortality [38].

Though Tharakan et al. [39] reported 13% of 38 cases of strokes in the young had mitral valve prolapse, other centres in India have not shown such high incidence. Smoking as a RF for CVD has always been considered equivocal as some authors have found positive association [40] but others have not [41]. Most of the Indian studies do not show smoking as one of the important RF, but our study did show smoking (beedi or cigarette) as an important RF in young and elderly men [27].

Though high haematocrit (Hct) is considered one of the important RFs [42,43], it is not yet clear how the level of Hct alters cerebral metabolism in the ischemic tissue. Kiyohara et al. [44] reported that when Hct is reduced below 30% (in experimental models), anemic hypoxia results which may precipitate global ischemia. On the other hand, the EC/IC bypass study group concluded that severity of strokes was not different in subjects with high Hgb values against those with lower values [45]. We found low normal Hgb concentration as an important RF for cerebral infarction in the young. Similar findings are also reported from a Japanese rural community survey in Hisayama [46]. Thus the controversy on the precise role of Hgb/Hct and other plasmatic factors to cerebral haemodynamics have remained a matter of constant debate [47].

No consistent relationship has been found between elevated cholesterol levels and the risk of stroke [29–31] and recent prospective studies have failed to establish a positive correlation in Indian subjects [27].

Conclusion

On the basis of currently available hospital based information from prospective stroke studies, and in absence of National health services/registries, in developing countries, some general recommendations are desirable.

1. It is essential to initiate hypertension and stroke registries at all university medical college hospitals (including their associated primary health care centres) to collect baseline data.

2. When a dependable infrastructure in rural areas is available (e.g., family planning programmes, health education and vaccination drives for eradication of infectious diseases, etc.), it may be possible to obtain similar data for rural populations.

3a. *Primary Health Care Centres and community centres should be the base station for such surveys as urban data will not truly reflect national problems and priorities* [48].

3b. Adequate training of available medical manpower by organising symposia or seminars is mandatory to define and standardise the nomenclature of the hypertension programme. Such programmes should stress simple guidelines on diagnosis, immediate domiciliary medical care, and vocational rehabilitation.

4. Special research teams located at well equipped neuroscience laboratories should devote their time and resources to study unusual factors as identified or suspected in a particular community.

References

1. Adelman SM (1981) Stroke 12 (part II): 1–69; 1–87.
2. Fratiglioni L, Wayne ME, Schoenberg DG et al. (1983) Neuroepidemiology 2: 101–106.
3. Kurtzke JF (1985) In: Mcdowell FH et al. (eds.) Cerebrovascular Survey Report NINCDS/NIH Publ. Health Services, USA, pp. 1–34.
4. Nencini P, Inzitari D, Baruffi MC et al. (1988) Stroke 19: 977–981.
5. Abraham J, Rao PSS, Inbaraj SG et al. (1970) Stroke 1: 477.
6. Dalal PM (1982) Jpn. Circ. J. 46: 621–624.
7. Hatano S (1977) Jpn. Heart J. 18: 171–177.
8. Hatano S and Omae T (1982) In: Proceedings of the First Asian Pacific Symposium on Stroke. Jpn. Circ. J. 46.
9. Aho K, Harmsen P, Hatano S et al. (1980) Bull. WHO 58(1): 113–130.
10. Viryavejakul A (1982) Jpn. Circ. J. 614–618.
11. Dube BK and Omar JB (1965) Indian Med. Assoc. 45: 257–263.
12. Padmavati S, Dhar P, Malhotra A et al. (1963) J. Assoc. Physicians India 11: 356–366.
13. Devichand and Caroli RK (1961) J. Indian Med. Assoc. 36: 565–572.
14. Gupta PD, Bawa YS and Wahi PL (1965) Indian Heart J. 17: 57–63.
15. Bharucha EP and Umerjee RS (1962) Neurol. Madras 10: 137–149.
16. Naik BK, Rao PS, Saboo R (1966) Indian Heart J. 18: 37–44.
17. Misra SS, Misra RN, Aggarwal PS et al. (1967) J. Indian Med. Assoc. 48: 525–530.
18. Dalal PM (1979) In: Goldstein M et al. (eds.) Advances in Neurology, Raven Press, New York, pp. 339–348.
19. Bansal BC, Prakash C, Jain AL et al. (1973) Neurol. India 21: 11–18.
20. Venkatraman S, Bhargava S and Virmani V (1977) J. Assoc. Physicians India 22: 523–529.
21. Banerjee AK, Chopra JS and Sawhney BB (1973) Neurol. India 21: 19.
22. Dalal PM, Dalal KP and Saraf O (1986) In: Oda T et al. (eds.) Internal Medicine. Elsevier Science Publications BV, Amsterdam, pp. 121–124.
23. Kapoor S, Chopra JS, Chander K et al. (1972) Neurol. India 20: 50.
22. Schoenberg BS (1980) In: Rose FC (ed.) Clinical Neuroepidemiology. Pitman Medical Publ. Co. Ltd, Tunbridge Wells, UK, pp. 151–162.
25. Dalal PM and Dalal KP (1986) Jpn. Heart J. 27: 901–910.
26. Dalal PM, Dalal KP and Vyas AC (1989) Neuroepidemiology 8: 160–164.
27. Dalal PM et al. (1989) Stroke 20: 157.
28. Abraham J (1973) In: Spillane JD (ed.) Tropical Neurology. Oxford University Press, London, UK, pp. 86–91.
29. Chopra JS and Prabhakar S (1979) Acta Neurol. Scand. 60: 289–300.
30. Bansal BC, Prakash C, Arya R et al. (1978) Stroke 9: 137–139.

31. Agrawal JK, Somani PN and Katiyar BC (1976) Neurol. India 24: 125–133.
32. Bedi HK, Bomb BS, Devpura JC et al. (1974) J. Assoc. Physicians India 22: 829–831.
33. Sharma SC, Vijayan JP, Sheth NH et al. (1978) J. Neurol. Neurosurg. Psychiatry 41: 118–121.
34. Srinivasan K (1984) Stroke 15: 733–735.
35. Bansal BC, Gupta RR, Prakash C (1980) Jpn. Heart J. 21: 171–183.
36. Weibers DO (1985) Arch. Neurol. 42: 1106–1113.
37. Komachi Y, Iida M, Shimamoto T (1971) Jpn. Circ. J. 35(2): 189.
38. Abbot RD, Donahue RP, Macmohan SW et al. (1987) J.A.M.A. 257: 949–952.
39. Tharakan J, Ahuja CK, Manchanda SC et al. (1982) Acta Neurol. Scand. 66: 295–302.
40. Salonen JT, Puska P, Tuomilehto J et al. (1982) Stroke 13: 327–333.
41. Herman B, Leyten ACM, Van Luijk JM et al. (1982) Stroke 13: 334–339.
42. Kannel WB, Gordan T, Wolf PA et al. (1972) Stroke 3: 409–420.
43. Tohgi H, Yamanouchi H, Murakami M et al. (1978) Stroke 9: 369–374.
44. Kiyohara Y, Fujishima M, Ishitsuka T et al. (1985) Stroke 16: 835–840.
45. Wade JPH, Taylor DW, Barnett HJM et al. (1987) Stroke 18: 68–71.
46. Kiyohara Y, Ueda R, Hasuo Y et al. (1986) Stroke 17: 687–692.
47. Grotta JC, Manner C and Pettigrew LC (1986) Stroke 17: 811–817.
48. Sevagram Medico Friend Circle (1983) World Health Forum 4: 365.

Management of ischemic strokes

Frank M. Yatsu and James C. Grotta
Department of Neurology, University of Texas Medical School at Houston, Houston, TX 77030, USA

Introduction

Ischemic strokes are caused by either (1) thrombosis due to atherosclerosis, including artery-to-artery emboli, as from carotid artery plaques, (2) embolic strokes of cardiac origin, and (3) lacunar strokes due to arteriolar occlusion, most commonly due to hypertension leading to lipohyalinosis. Acute therapies of ischemic strokes are aimed at (a) minimizing ischemic brain damage and (b) preventing stroke recurrences. Because brain tissue is exquisitely vulnerable to ischemic insults as well as to secondary events provoked by reperfusion and ischemia, therapeutic attempts must be initiated as early as possible after the stroke, likely a matter of less than several hours. In addition, the terminal nature of penetrating cerebral arterioles limits the options to develop collateral circulation. As a result of this anatomic variation preventing measures which might otherwise provoke the development of collateral circulation in the path distal to occlusion, the affected peripheral circulation, the so-called 'ischemic penumbra', must be optimized to avert secondary ischemic damage. The ischemic penumbra is secondarily compromised by the release of various vasoactive compounds from blood elements, such as platelets and thromboxane A2, and from ischemic brain tissue, such as other prostaglandin metabolites.

As a result of these considerations, acute ischemic stroke therapy is directed towards (1) the thrombus, (2) improvement of collateral circulation, particularly in the 'ischemic penumbra', as noted above, (3) prevention of secondary metabolic events resulting from ischemia and reperfusion which can aggravate the ischemic insult in precipitating irreversible neuronal damage. Considerations to minimize recurrences of ischemic strokes are beyond the scope of this discussion, but for atherothrombotic brain infarction they relate to use of antiplatelet agents and anti-atherosclerosis measures, particularly in reducing serum cholesterol, as reflected in low density lipoproteins (LDL) and increasing high density lipoproteins (HDL). For embolic strokes of cardiac origin, use of anticoagulation or antiplatelet agents should be considered and for lacunar strokes, control of hypertension and risk factors of atherosclerosis are critical to preventing recurrences.

Thrombus therapy

Although current studies have not been concluded to advise on the value and indications for thrombolytic agents, particularly tissue plasminogen activator (tPA), use of tPA or streptokinase, where available, may on occasion be justified when an acute thrombus is suspected and no hemorrhagic changes in brain are present. Animal experiments using autologous thrombi are dramatic in demonstrating angiographically proven recanalization with tPA, and results from the use of tPA and of streptokinase in myocardial infarction due to thrombosis are equally persuasive on the beneficial aspects of thrombolysis to promote reperfusion and preservation of ischemically impaired tissue. On the basis of anecdotal evidences so far, such as our own, early use of thrombolytic agents can be dramatic in preserving at-risk tissue and warrants consideration in the proper patient with acute ischemic strokes. Use of low molecular weight heparinoids offer another potentially useful therapy, now under study.

Since platelet hyperaggregability is present with acute ischemic strokes, particularly ABIs and embolic strokes of cardiac origin, use of antiplatelet agents is justified, such as aspirin or ticlopidine, although no prospective study has been undertaken to date to prove its efficacy acutely. Use of anticoagulation acutely, as with heparin, has not been proven to be of value so far for ischemic strokes despite the occurrence of thrombosis. Nonetheless, if a question of neurological progression is present, not attributable to edema, anticoagulation acutely is justified, particularly in the vertebrobasilar circulation. In these patients, we recommend that heparin be given without bolusing and that doses of 800–1,000 units per hour be infused intravenously to raise the partial thromboplastin time by 1.5 to 2.0 times control values. In addition, since cow derived heparin is associated with higher incidences of paradoxical thrombus formation, due to its inhibition of platelet prostacyclin synthesis, porcine heparin is recommended.

Collateral circulation and the 'ischemic penumbra'

Efforts to improve collateral circulation and 'ischemic penumbra' have concentrated on (a) improving hemorheological factors, (b) enhancing vasodilatation, and (c) maximizing the 'perfusion pressure'.

Hemorheological factors

The three major factors contributing to blood viscosity are erythrocyte deformability, hematocrit, and fibrinogen. To improve erythrocyte deformability, pentoxifylline (Trental) has been successful in the peripheral vascular circulation, but with acute ischemic stroke, its value occurred during the first several days following stroke, when the drug was given intravenously. The reason for oral dosing of pentoxifylline losing any benefits could not be explained, but the question whether intravenous dosing is more effective in reducing erythrocyte deformability and in improving hemorheological parameters more consistently is raised. Nonetheless, on the basis of benefits from intravenous pentoxifylline in significantly conveying neurological improvement compared to controls combined with its dramatic value in peripheral vascular disease, its use can be recommended in patients who display incomplete paralysis, reflecting the possibility of improvement. In addition, reports indicate that its use may decrease stroke recurrences, presumably by improving the hemorheological characteristics of stroke-prone patients, but further studies are needed for chronic therapy with this drug.

Viscosity reduction may yet be a useful adjunct in acute strokes, the studies have not demonstrated its value. In addition, the need to monitor patients for cardiac failure, fluid volume and cardiac output exceeds the likely therapeutic gains. Nevertheless, occasional patients with evidences of high blood viscosity, suggested by elevated hematocrit and increased fibrinogen concentrations, may benefit from either isovolemic or hypervolemic hemodilution. Since the latter may provoke cardiac failure, particularly in patients with known cardiac disease, and therefore require monitoring of pulmonary wedge pressures and cardiac output, isovolemic hemodilution is preferable. With this technique, essentially equal volumes of extracted blood are replaced with a volume expander, such as albumin, pentastarch or hetastarch. The 'ideal' hematocrit which maximizes both oxygen delivery and viscosity reduction is between 30–33%.

Therapies to reduce fibrinogen selectively using the snake venom ancrod have not been uniformly successful, and it cannot be recommended.

Vasodilators

Various vasodilators have not unequivocally caused improvement, although calcium channel blockers may convey its benefits through enhancement of vasodilation. Whether a stable analog of prostacyclin, a powerful vasodilator and platelet antiaggregant will be helpful, will require prospective studies on its effects. For reasons noted below, calcium channel blockers can be recommended for acute strokes because of its presumed effect in preventing cellular influx of calcium, both to the vascular muscles modulating tone but also neuronal cells. On the basis of its greater action on cerebral vessels, the dihydropyridine, nimodipine, may be more effective than the other calcium channel blockers.

Perfusion pressure

To optimize perfusion pressure, defined as the difference between the mean arterial and mean venous (or CSF) pressures, in order to maximize delivery of nutrients to neural cells and carry away metabolic wastes is problematic since arterial elevation may provoke hemorrhage or possibly brain edema. Nonetheless, on occasion, mild (15–20%) elevation of systemic blood pressure may be warranted, particularly when the mean arterial pressure is low, that is, below 100 mmHg. On the contrary, reduction of blood pressure when elevated is not indicated, unless hypertensive encephalopathy is a concern, a clinical diagnosis in which encephalopathy, diastolic blood pressures of over 140 mmHg and hemorrhages and edema of the fundi are usual.

Secondary metabolic effects

Modern neurochemical studies have shed light on a vast array of complex metabolic consequences of both ischemia and reperfusion which have detrimental effects on ischemic brain in aggravating ischemia and provoking ischemic brain damage. These factors relate to calcium ion entry into ischemic cells, which may be the crucial event in precipitating ischemic damage; free radical formation; release of excitotoxins which stimulate neurons and cause calcium influx; edema formation; and lactic acidosis.

Experimental studies are underway both in animal models of strokes and in patients on the value of drugs affecting these various metabolic events, but the single therapy which has been shown to avert ischemic brain damage is the use of calcium channel blockers. Although this compound may also increase blood flow in the ischemic tissue as well, its most dramatic effect appears to be in preventing calcium influx. As a result of these findings in humans, this drug can be recommended for acute ischemic strokes. Lactic acidosis may have damaging effects on cellular functions at certain reductions of pH; improving cerebral blood flow and minimizing ischemia are the best interventions since changing blood pH with bicarbonates will not affect intraneuronal pH. On the basis of studies using excitotoxin inhibitors, including the N-Methyl-D-Aspartate receptor, and their effectiveness on occasion in animals, human studies are currently planned. Use of this drug should await these investigations since untoward side effects may become a contraindication for human usage.

Newer studies on the value of 21-aminosteroids and of superoxide dismutase in reducing the damaging effects of free radicals offer tremendous optimism for future therapies in patients with acute ischemic strokes. Similarly, exciting results on the benefits of ganglioside which acts as a protective substrate also supports the hope for additional therapies in protecting ischemic brain.

Summary

In acute ischemic strokes, the three factors contributing to ischemic brain damage are the nature and character of the offending thrombus, the adequacy of the collateral circulation or 'ischemic penumbra', and the exquisite vulnerability of ischemic neurons to ischemic injury, particularly to secondary metabolic effects of ischemia. Efforts to treat each of these areas are justified if they can be initiated reasonably early following the ischemic stroke. For thrombus formation, acute use of thrombolytic agents is warranted if it is readily available and no brain hemorrhage is present. Aspirin or ticlopidine may also reduce progression, but are effective in preventing recurrences in ABIs. To improve cerebral blood flow, use of pentoxifylline is justified intravenously, and, on occasion, elevation of blood pressure modestly when low are warranted. For secondary metabolic effects, currently available calcium channel blockers can be used to avert calcium influx. Although multi-modal therapy affecting the thrombus, collateral circulation, and secondary metabolic factors provoking ischemic neuronal damage has not been proven, their use appears warranted on the basis of experimental and clinical studies.

References

1. Biller J et al. (1989) A dose escalation study of ORG 10172 (low molecular weight heparinoid) in stroke. Neurology 39: 262–265.
2. Del Zoppo GJ et al. (1986) Thrombolytic therapy in stroke: Possibilities and hazards. Stroke 17: 595–607.
3. Duke RJ et al. (1988) Intravenous heparin for the prevention of stroke progression in acute partial stable stroke: A randomized controlled trial. Ann. Int. Med. 105: 203–207.
4. Gelmers HJ et al. (1988) A controlled trial of nimodipine in acute ischemic stroke. N. Engl. J. Med. 318: 203–207.
5. Grotta JC (1987) Current medical and surgical therapy for cerebrovascular disease. N. Engl. J. Med. 317: 1505–1516
6. Hall E et al. (1988) 21-aminosteroid lipid peroxidation inhibitor U74006F protects against cerebral ischemia in gerbils. Stroke 19: 997–1002.
7. Hemodilution in Stroke Study Group (1989) Hypervolemic hemodilution treatment of acute stroke. Stroke 20: 317–323.
8. Imaizumi S et al. (1989) Superoxide dismutase activities and their role in focal cerebral ischemia. J. Cereb. Blood Flow Metab. 9(1): S217.
9. Italian Acute Stroke Study Group (1988) Haemodilution in acute stroke. Lancet 1: 318–321.
10. Jamieson DG et al. (1989) Ganglioside (GM1) treatment of acute ischemic infarction: A randomized, double-blind study using positron emission tomography. Neurology 39(1): 217.
11. Pentoxifylline Study Group (1987) Pentoxifylline in acute ischemic stroke. Stroke 18: 298.
12. Rothman SM and Olney JW (1986) Glutamate and the pathophysiology of hypoxic-ischemic brain injury. Ann. Neurol. 19: 105–111.
13. Yatsu FM et al. (1988) Anticoagulation of embolic strokes of cardiac origin: An update. Neurology 38: 314–316.

Part Two

Chronic Cerebrovascular Disease

Vascular dementia: Terminology and classification

Carlo Loeb
Institute of Neurology, University of Genova, Genova, Italy

Introduction

Vascular dementia (VD) is currently considered the second cause of dementia after the senile dementia of Alzheimer type (DAT) (Table 1).

Six criteria should be used to classify diseases: aetiology, clinical features, involved organ(s) or anatomy, stage monitored at follow-up, pathology and pathophysiology [1].

A classification based on aetiology is obviously the ideal one, although frequently impossible as, in fact, the case with VD. Moreover, a classification of VD based on brain pathology or on mixed clinical-pathological features seems fraught with further difficulties.

Actually, according to Tomlinson [2] any pathological process, including the vascular one, can produce dementia when it destroys a given amount of cerebral substance, about 100 ml. However, some patients with dementia had multiple small-sized infarctions [3] with apparently minimal parenchymal destruction.

Quite recently Scheinberg [4] emphasised a crucial point already widely discussed by others [2,5–7]: neither CT and/or MRI findings nor pathological evidence of infarction can necessarily mean that these cerebral vascular lesions are responsible for a state of dementia.

The aim of the present assessment of VD is to provide some support to the clinical investigators mainly in terms of comparable terminology, diagnostic and pathological criteria, without presuming to achieve the definitive classification.

Terminology

The criteria whereby dementia is defined are those of the DSM III R and should be regarded as tentative and provisional [8].

The label 'arteriosclerotic dementia' generously attached in the past to patients with intellectual impairment thought to be of vascular origin was substituted, in the literature after 1974, by the term 'multi-infarct dementia' (MID) [9].

Nonetheless multi-infarcts (MI) constitute but a part, however large, of dementia due or associated to vascular causes [10]. Therefore, the term vascular dementia

Table 1. Types of dementia in pathological studies

Authors	No. of cases	DAT N (%)	MID N (%)	MIX N (%)	Others and undefined N (%)
Corsellis [43]	89	30 (34)	42 (47)	17 (19)	–
Sourander & Sjogren (90)	258	132 (51)	72 (28)	–	54 (21)
Todorov et al. [91]	675	206 (31)	123 (18)	241 (36)	105 (15)
Jellinger [62]	1009	527 (52)	225 (22)	136 (14)	121 (12)
Tomlinson [2]	73	38 (52)	12 (16.5)	12 (16.5)	11 (15)
Molsa et al. [13	58	28 (48)	11 (19)	6 (10)	13 (23)
Wade et al. [44]	65	38 (59)	10 (15)	6 (9)	11 (17)
Totals	2227	999 (45)	495 (22)	418 (19)	315 (14)

seems more appropriate to identify conditions of intellectual impairment due to vascular origin.

Evaluation of the criteria to be used for classification

Clinical features and diagnostic criteria

The clinical criteria for the diagnosis of vascular dementia are reported in Table 2 [11].

The first discriminating diagnostic step is represented by the Hachinski's Ischemic Score (IS). In neuropathological series [12,13] the sensitivity and specificity of IS exceeded 70%. Purely clinical diagnostic criteria yielded, in various neuropathological series, a diagnostic accuracy of about 85% [14,15], showing that the combination of detailed medical, neurological, neuropsychological examinations, along with CT and MRI investigations, has a higher clinical diagnostic accuracy [16–19] (Table 3).

Table 2. Clinical criteria for the diagnosis of VD

1. Identification of a dementia syndrome (history, neurological examination, psychiatric interview, neuropsychological tests).
2. Exclusion of causes of dementia other than DAT and VD
3. Differential diagnosis between DAT and VD based on:
   - IS (equal or higher than 7)
   - MIS (equal or higher than 5; CT and MRI single or multiple low density areas or bright lesions)
   - Comparative evaluation of the clinical features ascribed to DAT and VD
   - Signs of BBB damage (increase in IgG index and albumin)
   - SEPs alterations
   - Focal EEG changes

Table 3. Sensitivity and specificity of the clinical diagnosis

Authors	No. of cases	Sensitivity %			Specificity %		
		AD	MID	MIX	AD	MID	MIX
Todorov et al. [91]	560	69	57	30	78	81	84
Jellinger [62]	1009	55	76	78	67	56	51
Molsa et al. [13]	58	71	73	17	73	77	92
Wade et al. [44]	65	87	17	50	78	93	70
Total	1692						

However, as O'Brien [20] rightly pointed out, the score does not seem to divide patients into a vascular and DAT group but rather into a large or medium sized infarct group and 'everything else'. The 'everything else' group includes, among others, patients with lacunas, Binswanger's disease, and particularly patients with mixed forms. A Modified Ischemic Score (MIS) [16] simply supplements the clinical data of the IS including a CT visualisation of the clinically postulated ischemic or lacunar infarctions, MRI further increases this possibility with its greater sensitivity in detecting small focal ischemic lesions in the deep white matter [21–23].

In spite of all these tests, at least approximately 30% of the patients may turn out to bear wrong diagnostic labels, especially those with mixed forms.

Anatomic distribution of the brain damage

Some studies attach great relevance to the location of the vascular lesion in producing dementia.

In particular, dementia is associated with bilateral thalamic lesions [24] with lesions located in the thalamus of the dominant hemisphere [25,26] or with lesions of both thalamic and cortical areas supplied by the middle cerebral artery [27–29].

The cortical-subcortical categorisation of dementia is still controversial [30–33].

Nevertheless, cortical and subcortical MIDs seem to differ in several respects regarding their clinical features, the occurrence of cardiac disease and finally, the mean total volume of infarctions (45 ml in cortical vs. 4 ml in subcortical MIDs) [3].

The distinction between cortical and subcortical MID is still an open question, but the distinction of vascular dementia according to the involved areas of the brain seems useful, especially concerning the prognosis [34]. White matter lesions deserve special mention: White matter lucencies or leuko-araiosis (LA) [35] appear with high frequency in VD patients but also in DAT patients and in age and sex-matched controls [36,37]. This neuroimaging feature correlates with the presence of mental impairment and with focal neurological deficits [38,39] and has been reported in the lacunar state and in Binswanger's disease [21,40–42]. More-

Table 4. Anatomic distribution of the vascular lesions in patients with dementia

1. Cortical (large or small infarctions)
2. Subcortical (small deep infarctions: thalamus, basal ganglia and surrounding white matter)
3. White matter (hypoperfusion, incomplete infarctions)
4. Diffuse (distribution as 1-2-3 in different association)

over, the histopathologically verified white matter changes have been attributed to hypoperfusion and explained as incomplete infarctions, being, at least in part, observed on CT and MRI [37]. The anatomic distribution of the lesions is listed in Table 4.

Clinical course and duration of survival (temporal profile)

The time of onset is difficult to ascertain owing to inaccuracies of both the observer and the patients or their families.

In neuropathological studies vascular dementia affects younger age groups than DAT [5,43,44], the respective mean age being 66.5 vs. 73.7 years. Mixed forms have a more delayed onset than DAT (74.9 years).

In clinical studies [15,45] global life expectancies were greater in DAT patients than in MID ones. However, MID patients have been noted to survive longer after becoming demented than patients with DAT [44]. Nonetheless, it is still uncertain whether VD really earns poorer prognosis than DAT, as pointed out by Mirsen and Hachinski [34].

The mixed forms have the shortest survival time [15,43,44].

Neuropathological lesions

Pathologically verified ischemic lesions occurring as the only alterations associated with dementia are listed in Table 5 (see references for [10]).

Some clinico-pathological entities deserve mention

(i) Subcortical arteriosclerotic encephalopathy (SAE) or Binswanger's disease (BD)

SAE had been considered an extremely rare condition until a few years ago. Patients with a typical SAE usually suffer from persistent arterial hypertension and show small infarcts or lacunae in their basal ganglia, thalamus and pons and an evolving clinical picture characterised by dementia, parkinsonism, pseudobulbar palsy, and urinary incontinence [64,65]. On the other hand, some patients with only a lacunar state have a clinical picture described as typical for SAE [66].

Moreover, it should be recalled that the clinical picture of some patients with neuropathological findings typical of SAE, was shown to be grossly at variance

Table 5. Neuropathological features and underlying mechanisms causing cerebral damage

1. Multiple large and/or small infarctions	Embolisation from the heart or atherosclerotic plaques in supraaortic vessels
2. Multiple lacunae (lacunar state)	Arteriolar, capillary arteriosclerosis; lypo-hyalinosis (small vessel disease)
3. Subcortical arteriosclerotic encephalopathy (SAE) or Binswanger's disease (BD)	
4. Watershed or borderzone infarction	Thrombosis or embolisation; showers of microemboli; 'misery perfusion syndrome', haemorheological alterations
5. Inflammatory angiopathies	Cerebral vasculitis due to different aetiologies
6. Aneurysms, arterio-venous malformations, subarachnoid hemorrhage	Compression of the circulatory pathways of the CSF; diffuse intra- and extracerebral bleedings, secondary hydrocephalus
7. Anoxic damage (acute or chronic): necrosis in the borderzone between contiguous cerebral arterial districts or diffuse necrosis (for references see [10])	Cardiac and/or respiratory failure due to different causes

with the classical one, in particular, their status was conspicuous for the absence of: any clinical sign (asymptomatic cases) [67,68]; any neurological sign [22,42,69]; any sign of dementia [67,68,70,71]; or any trace of hypertension [72], possibly owing to reduced cardiac output in the preterminal phase (from a few months to a few years) [68].

Binswanger's disease, a pure neuropathological diagnosis until a few years ago, came to be diagnosed 'in vivo' by means of CT [40,41,64,68,73–78] and/or MRI imaging [21,22,42,79–83].

Some authors stress ischaemia as the main pathophysiological process, not unlike MID [67,71] or other vascular forms of subcortical dementia [78]. The apparent conclusion is that the pathological lesions leading to SAE are probably due to ischaemia but they are not necessarily accompanied by dementia.

(ii) a) Inflammatory diseases of blood vessels (inflammatory angiopathies)
b) Haematological disorders

a) The mental disturbances occurring in cases with inflammatory angiopathy or vasculitis are almost always represented by confusional states which should be distinguished from true dementias.

Several aetiologies such as bacterial, viral, autoimmune, connective, fungal, parasitic, and miscellaneous causes (radiation, chemical, sarcoidosis) can be held responsible for vasculitis. Other less usual vascular diseases are moya-moya and fibromuscular dysplasia [6,46].

Vasculitis includes pathological changes of the vessel wall, with narrowing and occlusion of the vessel lumen, thrombosis with subsequent infarctions and, rarely, haemorrhages.

Although a rare disease, vasculitis due to several aetiologies perhaps represents one of the most frequently unsuspected derangements involving the brain vessels, bringing about neurological complications and, in rare cases, mental deterioration.

Mental deterioration and dementia may occur in the following diseases or syndromes: the aortic bifurcation syndrome [47–49]; giant cell arteritis or granulomatous angiitis [50,51]; polyarteritis nodosa, which may affect the CNS in 9% to 60% of cases [50,52,53]; lupus erythematosus, which shows neurological complications in up to 80% of cases, of which 28% exhibit psychiatric disturbances [54] and, in a few cases (5% of all cases with CNS involvement, [55]) a real state of dementia; rheumatic encephalopathy, rarely showing gross infarctions or multi-infarctions [56], primary cerebral amyloid angiopathy, showing deposition of amyloid in large and medium sized cerebral arteries leading to haemorrhages and red softenings, associated with senile plaques and neurofibrillary tangles [57]. The relationship with Alzheimer's disease is still unclear [58,59], as well as its association with rheumatoid vasculitis [60] and demyelinating disorders [61,62].

b) Hematologic disorders include disorders of the red blood cells (polycythaemia, sickle cell anaemia) macroglobulinaemia, leukaemia, leading to occlusive and haemorrhagic brain lesions sometimes heralded by mental changes, usually organic brain syndromes and, in rare cases, proper dementias [6,48,63].

(iii) Aneurysms and arteriovenous malformations; subarachnoid haemorrhage
In cases with intracerebral aneurysms, intellectual deterioration syndrome can occur before as well as after the rupture of the aneurysm. A hydrocephalus causing dementia can be brought about by an aneurysm of the basilar artery or of the vein of Galen compressing the aqueduct or to an adhesive arachnoiditis, blocking CSF reabsorption. Mental disturbances could also be related to the diffuse intra- and extracerebral bleedings, often accompanied by areas of ischemic softening.

Arteriovenous malformations can bring about mental deterioration, with a frequency ranging from 10 to 50% of all cases.

Such a demential syndrome seems to be much more related to the size than to the location of the aneurysm, inasmuch as the more widespread the malformation, the more the cerebral circulation suffers, with attending cerebral atrophy (for references see Loeb [10]).

Conclusion

An aetiological classification of VD is, at present, unfeasible, even if the pathophysiology of the cerebral ischaemia and infarctions associated with MID have been exhaustively assessed by Meyer et al. [84].

Table 6. Vascular diseases associated with dementia

1. Multi-infarct dementia (MID)
2. Lacunar dementia (LD)
3. Association of infarcts and lacunes
4. Suprabulbar palsy
5. Subcortical arteriosclerotic encephalopathy or Binswanger's disease
6. Single watershed or borderline infarction
7. Acute, subacute or chronic diffuse anoxia (references in [10])
8. Inflammatory diseases of blood vessels; haematological disorders
9. Intracranial aneurysms, arterio-venous malformations, subarachnoid haemorrhage
10. Hereditary MI dementia [92]
11. Hereditary amyloid angiopathy with recurrent cerebral haemorrhage [93,94]

A classification based on clinical grounds should follow the steps outlined in Table 2, and simply offers a list of vascular diseases associated with dementia (Table 6).

The differential clinical diagnosis between VD and DAT can be achieved at an acceptable level of confidence, but it leaves the mixed forms undiagnosed thus always leaving open the possible coexistence of a degenerative type of dementia. It is a hope that the diagnosis of degenerative dementia can be achieved with a high specificity by olfactory neurons biopsy [85]. The neuropathological assessment of VD (Table 5) raises some crucial unresolved points: 1) the cause and effect relationship between the vascular lesion and dementia, 2) the relationship between small and/or lacunar multiple infarctions and dementia, 3) the problem of mixed forms.

Brain infarctions with destruction of brain tissue up to 100 ml in the absence of specific neuropathological markers of degenerative dementia or other factors, are considered as a cause of dementia [2]. A modest loss of cerebral substance (lower than 100 ml) does not allow one to relate the dementia to the vascular lesion with certainty, in view of the fact that quite normal elderly subjects may exhibit cerebral losses of that size. However, besides the quantitative aspect of the lesion other factors such as the location of the lesion (particularly in deep areas of the brain, thalamus and basal ganglia) and the occurrence of enlargement of the ventricles and subarachnoid spaces should be taken into account as possible causes of dementia [17,25–27,29,86].

The mixed forms are even more puzzling, since it is difficult to assess in a given case the weight of the different pathological lesions responsible for the state of dementia [87]. The clinical course of VD shows that survival is higher in DAT than in VD, in which mortality is higher [15] and age dependent, showing an increased mortality with advancing age [88].

The statement already made by different authors [4,6,7,89] that the aetiology of VB is multifactorial seems acceptable, owing to the very fact that apparently similar vascular lesions may or may not be associated with dementia.

References

1. Ad Hoc Committee (1975) Stroke 6: 565–616.
2. Tomlinson BE (1980) In: Roberts PJ (ed.) Biochemistry of Dementia. John Wiley & Sons Ltd, Chichester, pp. 15–52.
3. Erkinjuntti T (1987) Acta Neurol. Scand. 75: 391–399.
4. Scheinberg P (1988) Stroke 19: 1291–1299.
5. Tomlinson BE, Blessed B and Roth M (1970) J. Neurol. Sci. 11: 205–242.
6. Brust JCM (1983) In: Mayeux R and Rosen WG (eds.) The Dementias. Raven Press, New York, pp. 131–147.
7. Brust JCM (1988) Arch. Neurol. 45: 799–801.
8. McKhann G, Drachman D, Folstein M, Katzman R, Price D and Stadlan E (1984) Neurology 34: 939–944.
9. Hachinski VC, Lassen NA, Marshall J (1974) Lancet 2: 207–209.
10. Loeb C (1985) In: Vinken PJ, Bruyn GW and Klawans HL (eds.) Handbook of Clinical Neurology vol. 2. Elsevier, Amsterdam, pp. 353–369.
11. Loeb C (1988) Eur. Neurol. 28: 87–92.
12. Rosen WG, Terry RD, Fuld PA, Katzman R and Peck A (1980) Ann. Neurol. 7: 486–488.
13. Molsa PK, Paljarvi L, Rinne JO, Rinne UK, Sako E (1985) J. Neurol. Neurosurg. Psychiat. 48: 1085–1090.
14. Erkinjuntti T, Haltia M, Palo J, Sulkava R and Paetau A (1988) J. Neurol. Neurosurg. Psychiat. 51: 1037–1044.
15. Barclay LL, Zemcov A, Blass JP and Sansone J (1985) Neurology 35: 834–840.
16. Loeb C and Gandolfo C (1983) Stroke 14: 399–401.
17. Meyer JS, Judd BW, Tawaklna T, Rogers RL and Mortel KF (1988) J.A.M.A. 256: 2203–2209.
18. Erkinjuntti T, Ketonen L, Sulkava R, Sipponen J, Vuorialho M and Iivanainen M (1987) J. Neurol. Neurosurg. Psychiat. 50: 37–42.
19. Meyer JS, McClintic KL, Rogers RL, Sims P and Mortel KF (1988) J. Neurol. Neurosurg. Psychiat. 51: 1489–1497.
20. O'Brien MD (1988) Arch. Neurol. 45: 797–799.
21. Erkinjuntti T, Sipponen JT, Iivanainen M, Ketonen L, Sulkava R and Sepponen RE (1984) J. Comp. Assist. Tom. 8: 614–618.
22. Brant-Zawadski M, Fein G, Van Dyke C, Kiernan R, Davenport L and De Groot J (1985) A.J.N.R. 6: 675–682.
23. Hershey LA, Modic MT, Greenough PG and Jaffe DF (1987) Neurology 37: 29–36.
24. Castaigne P, Buge A, Cambier J, Escourolle R, Brunet P and Degos JD (1966) Revue Neurol. 114: 89–107.
25. Ladurner G, Iliff LD, Sager WD and Lechner H (1983) In: Mcycr JS, Lechner H, Reivich M and Ott E (eds.) Cerebral Vascular Disease IV: Proceedings of the World Federation of Neurology Int. Conference 11, Salzburg, Sept. 23–25, 1982. Excerpta Medica, Amsterdam, pp. 236–243.
26. Ladurner G and Bone G (1986) In: Lechner H, Meyer JS and Ott E (eds.) Cerebrovascular Disease: Research and Clinical Management. Elsevier Science Publ. Co. Inc., Amsterdam, pp. 163–172.
27. Kitigawa Y, Meyer JS, Tachibana H, Mortel KF and Rogers RL (1984) Stroke 15: 1000–1009.
28. Meyer JS (1986) In: Lechner H, Meyer JS, Ott E (eds.) Cerebrovascular Disease: Research and Clinical Management. Elsevier Science Publ. Co. Inc., Amsterdam pp. 173–181.
29. Loeb C, Gandolfo C and Bino G (1988) Stroke 19: 560–565.
30. Albert ML (1978) In: Katzman R, Terry RD and Bick KL (eds.) Alzheimer's Disease: Senile Dementia and Related Disorders. Raven Press, New York, pp. 173–180.
31. Mayeux R, Stern Y, Rosen J and Benson F (1983) Ann. Neurol. 14: 278–283.
32. Benson DF (1983) In: Mayeux R and Rosen GW (eds.) The Dementias. Raven Press, New York, pp. 185–194.
33. Huber SJ, Shuttleworth EC, Paulson GW, Bellchambers MJG and Clapp LE (1986) Arch. Neurol. 43: 392–394.

34. Mirsen T and Hachinski V (1988) In: Meyer JS, Lechner H, Marshall J and Toole JF (eds.) Vascular and Multi-infarct Dementia. Futura Publ. Co. Inc., Mount Kisco NY, pp. 61–75.
35. Hachinski V, Potter P and Merskey H (1987) Arch. Neurol. 44: 21–23.
36. Inzitari D, Diaz F, Fox A, Hachinski VC, Steingart A, Lau C, Donald A, Wade J, Mulic H and Merskey H (1987) Arch. Neurol. 44: 42–47.
37. Brun A and Englund E (1986) Ann. Neurol. 19: 253–262.
38. Steingart A, Hachinski VC, Lau C, Fox AJ, Diaz F, Cape R, Lee D, Inzitari D and Merskey H (1987) Arch. Neurol. 44: 32–35.
39. Steingart A, Hachinski VC, Lau C, Fox AJ, Foz H, Lee D, Inzitari D and Merskey H (1987) Arch. Neurol. 44: 36–39.
40. Rosenberg GA, Kornfeld M, Stovring J and Bicknell JM (1979) Neurology 29: 1102–1106.
41. Loizou LA, Kendall BE and Marshall J (1981) J. Neurol. Neurosurg. Psychiat. 44: 294–304.
42. Kinkel WR, Jacobs L, Polachini I, Bates V and Heffner RR Jr (1985) Arch. Neurol. 42: 951–959.
43. Corsellis JAN (1962) Mental Illness and the Aging Brain. Oxford University Press, London.
44. Wade JPH, Mirsen TR, Hachinski VC, Fisman M, Lau C and Merksey H (1987) Arch. Neurol. 44: 24–29.
45. Roth M (1955) J. Ment. Sci. 101: 281–301.
46. Zeek PM (1953) New Engl. J. Med. 248: 764–772.
47. Currier RD, DeJong RN and Bole GG (1954) Neurology 4: 818–830.
48. Aita JA (1964) Neurologic manifestations of general diseases. C.C. Thomas, Springfield, Ill.
49. Mumenthaler M (1984) In: Toole JF (ed.) Cerebrovascular disorders. 3rd edn. Raven Press, New York, pp. 299–312.
50. Bruetsch WL (1971) In: Minckler J (ed.) Pathology of the Nervous System. McGraw-Hill, New York, pp. 1456–1481.
51. Koo EH and Massey EW (1988) J. Neurol. Neurosurg. Psychiat. 51: 1126–1133.
52. Rose GA and Spencer H (1957) Q. J. Med. 26: 43–81.
53. Ford RG and Siekert GR (1965) Neurology 15: 114–122.
54. Tindal RSA (1980) In: Rosenberg RN (ed.) Neurology. Grune and Stratton, New York, pp. 41–77.
55. Devinsky O, Petito CK and Alonso DR (1988) Ann. Neurol. 23: 380–384.
56. Benda CE (1948) Arch. Neurol. Psychiat. 59: 262–264.
57. Okazaki H, Reagan TJ and Campbell RJ (1979) Mayo Clin. Proc. 54: 22–31.
58. Mandybur TI (1975) Neurology 25: 120–126.
59. Torack RM (1975) Am. J. Pathol. 81: 349–365.
60. Mandybur TI (1979) Neurology 29: 1336–1340.
61. Heffner RR, Porro RS, Olson ME and Earle KM (1976) Arch. Neurol. 33: 501–506.
62. Jellinger K (1976) Acta Neurol. Belg. 76: 83–102.
63. Logothetis J, Silverstein P and Coe J (1970) Arch Neurol. 3: 564–573.
64. Caplan LR and Schoene WC (1978) Neurology 28: 1206–1215.
65. Tomonaga M, Yamanouchi H, Tohgi H and Kameyama M (1982) J. Am. Geriatr. Soc. 30: 524–529.
66. Nichols FT III and Mohr JP (1986) In: Barnett HJM, Mohr JP, Stein BM and Yatsu FM (eds.) Stroke. Pathophysiology, Diagnosis and Management, vol. 2. Churchill Livingstone, New York, pp. 875–885.
67. De Reuck J, Crevits L, De Coster W, Sieben G and Van Eecken H (1980) Neurology 30: 920–928.
68. Lotz PR, Ballinger WE and Quisling RG (1986) A.J.R. 147: 1209–1214.
69. Burger PC, Burch JG and Kunze U (1976) Stroke 7: 626–631.
70. Olszewski I (1962) World Neurol. 3: 359–375.
71. Huang K, Wu L and Luo Y (1985) Can. J. Neurol. Sci. 12: 88–94.
72. Tanaka M, Ikuta F and Oyake Y (1969) Clin. Neurol. 9: 398–405.
73. Valentine AR, Moseley IF and Kendall BE (1980) J. Neurol. Neurosurg. Psychiat. 43: 139–142.
74. Zeumer H, Schonsky B and Sturm KW (1980) J. Comp. Assist. Tom. 4: 14–19.
75. Goto K, Ishii N and Fukasawa H (1981) Radiology 141: 687–695.
76. Loizou LA, Jefferson JM and Smith WT (1982) J. Neurol. Neurosurg. Psychiat. 45: 409–417.

77. Suzuki T, Takahashi S, Kashiwaba M et al. (1985) J. Neurol. 232 (suppl): 302.
78. Roman GC (1987) J.A.M.A. 258: 1782–1788.
79. Besson JAO, Corrigan FM, Iljon Foreman E and Ashcroft GW (1983) Lancet 2: 789.
80. Bradley WG, Waluch V, Brant-Zawadzki M et al. (1984) Noninvasive Med. Imaging 1: 35–41.
81. Dougherthy JH, Simmonds JD and Parker J (1986) Stroke 17: 146.
82. George AE, De Leon MJ, Kalnin A et al. (1986) A.J.N.R. 7: 567–570.
83. Zimmerman RD, Fleming CA, Lee BCP et al. (1986) A.J.R. 146: 443–450.
84. Meyer JS, McClintic K, Sims P, Rogers RL and Mortel KF (1988) In: Meyer JS, Lechner H, Marshall J and Toole JF (eds.) Vascular and Multi-infarct Dementia. Futura Publ. Co. Inc., Mount Kisco, NY, pp. 129–147.
85. Talamo BR, Rudel RA, Kosik KS, Lee Vm-Y, Neff S, Adelman L and Kanner JS (1989) Nature 337: 736–739.
86. Marshall J (1988) In: Meyer JS, Lechner H, Marshall J, Tole JF (eds.) Vascular and Multi-infarct Dementia. Futura Publ. Co. Inc., Mount Kisco NY, pp. 1–3.
87. Ulrich J, Probst A and Wuest M (1986) J. Neurol. 233: 118–122.
88. Lechner H, Bertha G and Ott E (1988) In: Meyer JS, Lechner H, Marshall J and Toole JF (eds.) Vascular and Multi-infarct Dementia. Futura Publ. Co. Inc., Mount Kisco, NY, pp. 101–111.
89. Tomlinson BE (1977) In: Wells CE (ed.) Dementia. F.A. Davis Co., Philadelphia, pp. 113–153.
90. Sourander P and Sjogren H (1970) In: Wolstenholme GE and O'Connor M (eds.) Alzheimer's Disease and related Conditions. Churchill, London, pp. 11–32.
91. Todorov AB, Go RCP, Constantinidis J and Elston RC (1975) J. Neurol. Sciences 26: 81–98.
92. Sourander P and Walinder J (1977) Acta Neuropath. Berl. 39: 247–254.
93. Gudmundsson G, Hallgrimsson J, Jonasson TA and Biarnason O (1972) Brain 95: 387–404.
94. Wattendorf AR, Bots Th AM, Went LN and Endtz LJ (1982) J. Neurol. Sci. 55: 121–135.

Pharmacological treatment of multi-infarct dementia

Maynard M. Cohen, Leyla de Toledo-Morrell and Frank Morrell
Department of Neurological Sciences, Rush-Presbyterian-St. Luke's Medical Center, 1653 W. Congress Parkway, Chicago, IL 60612, USA

Introduction

Dementia secondary to cerebral infarction is generally considered to follow ischemic destruction of 100 ml or more of tissue [1,2] or involvement of specific anatomic structures, such as the mesial temporal lobe, mammillary bodies, thalamus, subthalamic region, mesencephalon or basal forebrain [3,4,]. The hippocampal formation, in particular, has been implicated as being critical for recent memory in experimental animals and in humans [5–8]. Bilateral hippocampal lesions disrupt spatial memory or cognitive mapping in lower mammals [6] and lead to rapid loss of newly acquired information [9,10]. Humans with left temporal lobe dominance for speech who have sustained damage to the left hippocampus and parahippocampal gyrus exhibit impaired learning and recall of verbal information. Similar lesions to identical structures on the right affects memory for non-verbal material, such as spatial localization and abstract pictures [7].

The hippocampus is particularly sensitive to episodes of hypoxia and global cerebral ischemia as well as to local interruption of its blood supply. This sensitivity is demonstrated clinically in those patients exhibiting amnesia [10,11] and pathological evidence of hippocampal damage after experiencing cardiac arrest [8,12]. Ischemic hippocampal necrosis is a delayed rather than acute event in both experimental animals and in humans. Petito et al. [12] noted that eight patients dying 18 hours or less after cardiac arrest exhibited only mild damage in the hippocampus and moderate alterations in the putamen as well as in the border zone cortex and insular cortex. Severe alterations were present in all four areas, however, in those six patients surviving 24 hours or longer.

In addition to delayed hippocampal alterations as a consequence of cardiac arrest, there is evidence that some metabolic changes persist in ischemic areas of the brain for extensive periods after the initial insult has terminated [13,14]. Patients with multi-infarct dementia have also been noted to exhibit a diminished vaso-responsiveness to the inhalation of oxygen compared to individuals with Alzheimer's disease or to normal controls [15].

Decline in cerebral function and metabolism with aging as well as the co-existence of other cerebral degenerative disease may contribute to the dementia associated with multiple areas of cerebral infarction. Aged rats have been noted to demonstrate greater declines in cerebral high energy phosphates following ischemia than young mature controls [16], as well as decline in certain aspects of recent memory [17]. Clinical and pathological studies revealed as many as 40% of demented patients to have symptoms of dementia secondary to a combination of vascular events and degeneration of the Alzheimer type [4].

The persistence of adverse or deficient metabolic activity that could be counteracted to some extent by pharmacological therapy, the experimental evidence that some memory loss secondary to the aging process can be alleviated by the use of drugs, a report of improved cognition after control of risk factors for multi-infarct dementia [18], and positive findings in some preliminary clinical studies indicate that benefits may be obtained by treating certain forms of multi-infarct dementia with pharmacological agents.

Three forms of treatment have been hypothesized to yield clinical benefits by interfering with the pathogenetic mechanisms underlying organic dementia [19]: (1) Arterial vasodilatation to increase cerebral blood flow and secondarily improve cerebral metabolism; (2) agents directly supporting neuronal metabolism, and (3) modification of specific neuronal circuits.

A wide variety of drugs have received varying degrees of attention over the years. Most have been disappointing and clinical use, when it does occur, continues only because more effective agents have been lacking. The following agents are considered here either because recent reports of benefit have appeared in the literature, or animal studies have shown protection of hippocampal areas important for mnemonic function.

Cyclandelate

Blakemore [20] replicated a study of nearly two decades earlier, using the Hachinski scale [21] to aid in the selection of patients with dementia on the basis of multiple cerebral infarction. Three hundred and three patients, recruited by 78 general practitioners were treated with 1600 mg cyclandelate daily for 12 weeks. Significant improvement was noted in both the Blessed Dementia scale and the Parkside Behavioral Scale. Although no correlation was found between the pretreatment Hachinski Ischemia Score and improvement as measured by the dementia and behavioral scales, increasing severity of ischemia during the study period was related to a lack of significant improvement in the Blessed and Parkside Scales.

Dihydroergotoxine mesylate (DEM, Hydergine®)

Although DEM is presently one of the most commonly employed drugs for the treatment of dementia in the aged, controversy still exists as to its therapeutic efficacy [22]. Yoshikawa et al. [23] studied 550 patients with cognitive and neurological deficits secondary to cerebrovascular disease. Patients received daily doses of DEM of either 3 mg sublingually or 6 mg orally. Improvement of behavioral symptoms of a moderate or better degree was noted in 17.9% of patients on the lower dose. Those symptoms included problems in concentration, memory deficits, and loss of vigor. Patients receiving 6 mg daily, however, exhibited improvement at the rate of 48.9%.

Bromocriptine

Since patients with multi-infarct dementia often exhibit loss of initiative, apathy, bradykinesia, and impairment of other aspects of frontal lobe function, Nadeau and his associates [24] considered the possibility that those clinical findings might be related to ischemic destruction of projections from midbrain dopaminergic neurons to the striatum, mesolimbic structures and frontal cortex. They also noted that therapy with bromocriptine had been reported to result in improvement in a patient with akinetic mutism from hypothalamic damage [25] and in another with progressive supranuclear palsy [26]. When they treated seven individuals with vascular dementia with the same drug, however, neuropsychological testing failed to exhibit any benefit and performance worsened for several patients while on the drug.

Piracetam (2-oxo-1-pyrrolidine-acetamide)

Although Piracetam is a cyclic derivative of GABA, it has none of the pharmacological properties or physiological activities of GABA. This drug has been reported to improve verbal learning in young healthy volunteers following 14 days administration of 1.6 g/day [27]. However, its effect in patients with impairment of mentation secondary to cerebral infarction has not been demonstrated. Moreover, piracetam failed to produce any significant effect on regional cerebral blood flow by the Xenon inhalation technique in moderately demented patients [28]. The combination of piracetam with choline, however, has been reported as more effective than either compound alone in restoring memory loss in aged Fischer rats [29]. Platel et al. [30] found retention of information in mice to be facilitated by intraperitoneal injection of 2000 mg/kg of piracetam. The same facilitation was achieved with 50 mg/kg of piracetam when accompanied by 50 mg/kg of choline. Choline alone, to the point of toxicity, was without effect.

Nimodipine

Certain calcium entry blockers have received considerable attention because of their ability to relieve the vasospasm second to the rupture of an intracranial aneurysm and to ameliorate ischemic neuronal damage [31,32].

Depolarization of the cell membrane secondary to ischemia allows a sudden influx of calcium into the intracellular compartment. The elevated calcium concentration interferes with oxidative phosphorylation in the mitochondria and consequently energy formation in the form of ATP is impaired [33]. The dihydropyridine calcium entry blocker, nimodipine, has been reported to significantly increase local cerebral blood flow in normal rats [34] as well as in dogs whose cerebral circulation had been restored after temporary ligation of the aorta [35]. The neurological status of both dogs [35] and pigtailed monkeys [36] was improved compared to untreated animals when nimodipine was given either pre- or post-ischemia.

Mabe et al. [37] produced severe fore-brain ischemia in rats for 30 min by inducing mild hypotension after four vessel occlusion. Two hours after release of the occlusion the ATP level recovered to a significantly greater degree in those animals pretreated with nimodipine than in the control group. Recovery of electroencephalographic activity was also better in drug-treated animals. The authors suggested the results to be due either to improvement of postischemic hypoperfusion or to a direct action on metabolic processes during the reperfusion period.

Nimodipine has been reported to be effective in improving at least one measure of learning in aged rabbits. Deyo and his associates [38] noted that sufficient alteration in calcium ion homeostasis in aged subjects results in an increase in concentration of intra-cellular calcium which may influence learning by any of several mechanisms. They concluded that decreasing the influx of calcium ion could reduce prolonged calcium-activated currents or minimize calcium toxicity to neurons. They then noted that nimodipine accelerated associative learning in both young and aged rabbits as indicated by the more rapid acquisition of conditioned eye blinks.

Clinically, nimodipine has been reported to be effective in the treatment of acute cerebral ischemia as well as memory defects secondary to cerebral infarction. Gelmers et al. [39] treated 186 patients in a double-blind, placebo controlled trial of nimodipine for four weeks following an acute cerebral infarction. Patients were then followed for an additional six months. Mortality was reduced in the treatment group, but the benefit appeared limited to males. Those patients treated with nimodipine also exhibited a significantly better neurological outcome than did the control group, as assessed by the Mathew Scale of neurological deficit.

Bono et al. [40] reported on 32 patients followed for one year in a double blind, cross-over study. In the second phase 20 of the 32 were selected to continue on nimodipine in an open fashion. The nimodipine treated patients exhibited a significant improvement of verbal memory performance, using the Babcock I and II, and the digit span tests.

Pentoxifylline (Trental, 3,7,dimethyl-1-[5 oxohexyl]xanthine)

Pentoxifylline is a vaso-active phosphodiesterase inhibitor with effects on both peripheral vasculature and cerebral blood vessels. The drug has been demonstrated to increase peripheral circulation, decrease blood viscosity, inhibit platelet aggregation, and increase red cell deformability [41]. In 1974 Ganser and Boksay [42] reported pentoxifylline to reduce the cerebral edema secondary to freezing lesions in the cat.

Hartmann, Becker, and Cohen [43] demonstrated that this agent produced mitochondrial hypertrophy in cerebral neurons. The mitochondrial hypertrophy was most evident in the hippocampus, was restricted to neurons, and was of sufficient degree to result in an increase of mitochondrial mass. Since the mitochondrion is the site of oxidative phosphorylation, cerebral high energy phosphates were studied in relation to ischemia. When pentoxifylline was administered post-ischemia to experimental animals, concentrations of phosphocreatine and ATP were maintained in the brain at levels higher than in controls [41,44].

Spatial memory, and certain physiological parameters that are also associated with hippocampal activity have been noted to decline in aged rats. Reduced binding of cholinergic muscarinic receptors may occur in the aging process as well [45,46]. These behavioral, physiological, and anatomical findings may be reproduced to some extent when infarctive processes involve the hippocampus. The effects found in aging then bear a relationship to those observed in certain aspects of multi-infarct dementia.

Employing an 8 arm radial maze to test memory in Fischer rats, we demonstrated that pentoxifylline was indeed successful in reversing age-related deficits in spatial memory [47]. Since pentoxifylline was shown to improve energy metabolism in the face of cerebral ischemia, we considered that improved acetylation of choline (an energy requiring process) might result when pentoxifylline was administered together with choline. Addition of choline chloride failed to improve the accuracy of choice above that achieved by pentoxifylline alone, however.

Pentoxifylline also had beneficial effects on two electrophysiological measures of hippocampal synaptic plasticity which are intimately related to impairments in spatial memory loss, namely kindling and long term potentiation [48]. In the kindling paradigm a subthreshold electrical stimulus is applied briefly to a local brain area. Initially the stimulation results in only brief after-discharges (AD) and no behavior. With repeated stimulation on successive days, however, the AD gradually increases in duration and spreads to distant brain regions. A progressive alteration in behavior occurs, culminating in a major motor convulsion. Aged rats kindled via perforant path stimulation required nearly twice as many trials as young mature animals before reaching the kindling criterion [49]. Pentoxifylline-treated old animals, however, kindled significantly faster than did old saline controls (48).

Long term potentiation refers to an enhancement of synaptic transmission seen following brief trains of high frequency stimulation. In our experiments LTP was established in rats by stimulating the perforant path and recording from the dentate gyrus, using a procedure similar to that described by Barnes [50]. In accord with Barnes' findings [50], aged rats potentiated to the same extent as did the younger animals, however they lost the potentiated response at a much faster rate. Pentoxifylline-treated aged animals lost potentiation much more slowly than the age-matched saline controls [49]. The drug exerted no effect on the young in either behavioral or electrophysiological studies. Thus, these results taken together, indicate that a pharmacological manipulation which improves spatial memory in aged rats also augments hippocampal synaptic efficacy.

Dominguez [51] used the Hachinski Scale to select 30 patients for treatment of multi-infarct dementia with pentoxifylline. Twenty seven completed four months of treatment, and were considered to demonstrate significant improvement of impaired memory by the Barbizet test. The practical abilities of the patients were considered to be improved as demonstrated by the constructional apraxia test.

The potential benefits of pentoxifylline were evaluated by Parnetti et al. [52] in 60 elderly persons exhibiting clinical evidence of mental deterioration for less than 6 months. They reported that 400 mg of pentoxifylline administered three times daily significantly improved mnemonic function in these patients during treatment periods.

Propentofylline

Experimental evidence suggests that another xanthine derivative, propentofylline may be beneficial in ameliorating memory deficits secondary to ischemic insults involving the hippocampus. The carotid arteries of 81 Mongolian gerbils were occluded for 10 min and the intensity of Nissl staining in the Ca_1 neurons assessed densitometrically 4 days later. Even when propentofylline was administered 1 hour after the occlusion, Ca_1 neurons exhibited evidence of significant protection. No such benefit was obtained with the administration of phenobarbital [53].

Conclusion

Experimental investigations in animals and pathological studies in humans have highlighted the relationship of the hippocampus to the acquisition and retention of recent memory. The decline in recent memory in aging has also been demonstrated to be associated with alterations in hippocampal electrophysiology. Several pharmacological agents have been reported as successful in reversing the loss of short term memory in aged rats, and there is clinical evidence that these agents may be helpful to patients who have experienced memory deficits as a result of cerebral infarcts.

References

1. Tomlinson BE and Henderson G (1976) In: Terry RD and Gershon S (eds.) Neurobiology of Aging. Raven Press, New York, pp. 183–204.

2. Tomlinson BE, Blessed G and Roth M (1970) J. Neurol. Sci. 11: 205–242.
3. Scheinberg P (1988) Stroke 19: 1291–1299.
4. Katz DI, Alexander MP and Mandell AM (1987) Arch. Neurol. 44: 1127–1133.
5. Zola-Morgan S and Squire LR (1986) Behav. Neurosci. 100: 155–160.
6. Olton DS (1983) In: Siefert W (ed.) Neurobiology of the Hippocampus. Academic Press, London, pp. 335–373.
7. Milner B (1978) In: Buser PA and Rousel-Buser A (eds.) Symposium on Cerebral Correlates of Conscious Experience. Elsevier, Amsterdam.
8. Zola-Morgan S, Squire LR and Amaral DC (1986) J. Neurosci. 6: 2950–2967.
9. De Toledo-Morrell L, Geinisman Y and Morrell F (1988) In: Neural Plasticity. Alan R. Liss, New York, pp. 283–328.
10. Squire LR (1981) J. Neurol. Sci. 1: 635–640.
11. Volpe BT, Holtzman JD and Hirst W (1986) Neurology 36: 408–411.
12. Petito CK, Feldman E, Pulsinelli WA and Plum F (1987) Neurology 37: 1281–1286.
13. Cohen MM, Catanzaro R and Pocchiari F (1969) Proc. Internat. Soc. Neurochem. (Abstract).
14. Helpern JA, Martin GB, Quaday K, Paradis N, Nowak R and Welch K (1989) J. Cereb. Blood Flow Metab. 9 (suppl. 1): S720.
15. Judd BW, Meyer JS, Rogers RL, Gandhi S, Tanahashi N, Mortel KF and Tawaklna T (1986) J. Am. Geriatr. Soc. 34: 355–360.
16. Cohen MM, Kopp SJ, Pettegrew JW and Glonek T (1984) European Neurol. 23: 141–143.
17. De Toledo-Morrell L, Morrell F and Fleming S (1984) Behav. Neurol. Sci. 98: 902–907.
18. Meyer JS, Judd BW, Tawaklna T, Rogers RL and Mortel KF (1986) J.A.M.A. 256: 2203–2209.
19. Spagnoli A and Tognoni G (1983) Drugs 26: 44–69.
20. Blakemore CB (1987) Drugs 33 (suppl. 2): 110–113.
21. Hachinski VC , Iliff LD, Zihka E, Boulay GH, McAllister et al. (1975) Arch. Neurol. 32: 632–637.
22. Thienhaus OJ, Wheeler BG, Simon S, Zeman FP and Hartford JT (1987) J. Amer. Geriatr. Soc. 35: 219–223.
23. Yoshikawa M, Hirai S, Aizawa T, Kurojiwa S, Goto F, Sofue I, Toyokura Y, Yamamura H and Iwasaki Y (1983) J. Amer. Geriatr. Soc. 31: 1–7.
24. Nadeau SE, Malloy PF and Andrew ME (1988) Ann. Neurol. 24: 270–272.
25. Ross ED and Steward RM (1981) Neurology 31: 1435–1439.
26. Jackson JA, Jankovic J and Ford J (1983) Ann. Neurol. 13: 273–278.
27. Dimond SJ, Brouwers TM (1976) Psychopharmacology 49: 307–309.
28. Gustafson L, Risberg J, Johanson M, Fransson M and Maximilian VA (1978) Psychopharmacology 56: 115–117.
29. Bartus RT, Dean RL III, Sherman RA, Friedman E and Beer B (1981) Neurobiol. Aging 2: 3–8.
30. Platel A, Jalfre M, Pawelec C, Roux S and Porsolt RT (1984) Pharmacol. Biochem. Behav. 21: 209–212.
31. Farber L (1981) Life Sci. 29: 1289–1295.
32. Seisjo BK (1981) J. Cereb. Blood Flow Metab. 1: 155–185.
33. Nayler WG (1981) Am. J. Pathol. 102: 262–270.
34. Mohamed AA, Mendelow AD, Teasdale GM, Harper AM and McCulloch I (1985) J. Cereb. Blood Flow Metab. 5: 26–33.
35. Steen PA, Newberg LA, Milde JH and Michenfelder ID (1983) J. Cereb. Blood Flow Metab. 3: 38–43.
36. Steen PA, Gisvold SE, Milde JH, Newberg LA, Scheithauer BW, Lanier WL and Michenfelder JD (1985) Anesthesiol. 62: 406–414.
37. Mabe H, Nagai H, Takagi T, Umemura S and Ohno M (1986) Stroke 17: 501–505.
38. Deyo RA, Straube KT and Disterhoft JF (1989) Science 243: 809–811.
39. Gelmers KJ, Gorter K, de Weerdt CJ and Wiezer HJA (1988) N. Engl. J. Med. 318: 203–207.
40. Bono G, Sinfioriani E, Trucco M, Cavallini A, Acuto GC and Nappi G (1985) In: Betz E, Deck K, Hoffmeister F (eds.) Nimodipine – Pharmacological and Clinical Properties. Schattauer, Stuttgart, pp. 275–287.

41. Ward A and Clissold SP (1987) Drugs 34: 50–97.
42. Ganser V and Boksay I (1974) Neurology 24: 487–493.
43. Hartmann JF, Becker R and Cohen MM (1977) Neurology 27: 77–84.
44. Bluhm RE, Molnar J and Cohen MM (1985) Clin. Neuropharm. 8: 280–285.
45. De Toledo-Morrell L and Morrell F (1985) Ann. NY Acad. Sci. 444: 296–311.
46. Bartus RT, Dean RL, Beer B and Lippa AS (1982) Science 217: 408–416.
47. De Toledo-Morrell L, Morrell F, Fleming S and Cohen MM (1984) Behav. Neurol. Biol. 42: 1–8.
48. De Toledo-Morrell L, Geinisman Y and Morrell F (1988) Neurobiol. Aging 9: 581–590.
49. De Toledo-Morrell L, Morrell F and Fleming S (1984) Behav. Neurosci. 98: 902–907.
50. Barnes CA (1979) J. Comp. Physiol. Psychol. 93: 74–104.
51. Dominguez D (1986) In: Gotoh F and Lechner H (eds.) Haemorheology: A New Approach to Cerebrovascular Diseases. Royal Society of Medicine Services, London, pp. 20–23.
52. Parnetti L, Ciufetti G, Mercuri M, Lupattelli G and Senin U (1986) Pharmatherapeutica 4: 617–627.
53. DeLeo J, Schubert P and Kreutzberg GW (1988) Stroke 19: 1535–1539.

Cerebral blood flow and metabolism in chronic cerebrovascular disease with emphasis on the clinical use of CBF tomography by SPECT in vascular dementia

Niels A. Lassen and Gunhild Waldemar

Department of Clinical Physiology/Nuclear Medicine, Bispebjerg Hospital, DK-2400 Copenhagen NV, and Department of Neuromedicine, Rigshospitalet, DK-2100 Copenhagen Ø, Denmark

Introduction

Chronic cerebrovascular disease (CVD) is defined here as comprising all patients with chronic brain symptoms caused by diseases affecting the brain vessels. Two broad clinical categories are prominent. First, patients who have suffered severe focal neurological symptoms and often also dementia after a major stroke. Such chronic stroke cases are usually easy to diagnose accurately simply on the clinical evidence. Second, patients in whom progressive dementia is the all dominant clinical manifestation of the CVD. Such cases are generally called *Vascular Dementia* and they can be very difficult to distinguish clinically from cases of primar *Degenerative Dementia* such as Alzheimer's, or Pick's disease.

In this paper we will discuss the pathophysiology of chronic CVD in terms of the alterations of cerebral blood flow (CBF) and of cerebral metabolic rate of oxygen ($CMRO_2$). Emphasis will be put on the clinical value of adding such measurements to the classical neuroimaging techniques CT and MRI for the differential diagnosis between vascular and degenerative dementia.

CBF and $CMRO_2$ in CVD

In all chronic brain diseases with dementia, due to vascular disease or to other causes such as degenerative diseases, trauma or infection, *CBF and $CMRO_2$ are reduced in parallel.*

This was already shown for the senile dementias many years ago using the Kety-Schmidt inert gas technique for measuring average CBF and $CMRO_2$ of the whole brain, as exemplified in the study by Lassen et al. [1].

More recently it has also become possible to measure CBF and $CMRO_2$ *regionally* in the brain using positron emitting radioactive isotopes for tomographic imaging. Such studies have shown that in chronic stroke cases, months or years after the acute event, CBF and $CMRO_2$ are reduced proportionally in all brain

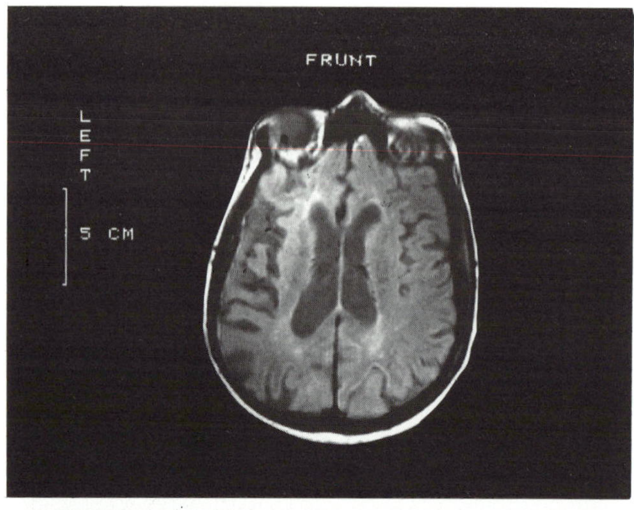

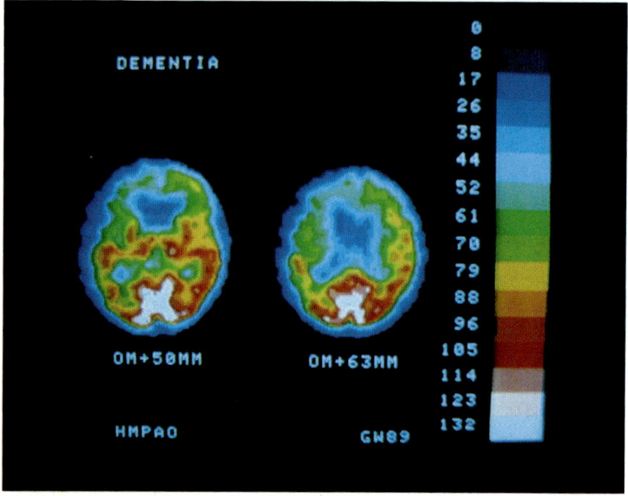

Fig. 1. Case of vascular dementia with single large cortical infarct in MCA-ACA teritory on left side. Above: MRI. Below: SPECT; note that the extension of the lesion exceeds that on MRI.

regions. This is true even if a vascular occlusion stills exists, e.g., an occlusion of the internal carotid artery. In other words, chronic stroke cases, even those with persisting arterial occlusion, do not suffer from persistent local oxygen lack (the so-called chronic ischemic penumbra) and will not, either clinically or with regard to CBF measured at rest, show any improvement by vascular surgery as in the form of an EC/IC by-pass.

The pattern of a proportional reduction in *regional* CBF and $CMRO_2$ was also found in a group of demented, elderly patients (average 65 years) reported by Frackowiak et al. [2]. These authors used positron emission tomography (PET) with radioactive oxygen-15 as the tracer and studied 9 cases of vascular dementia and 13 cases of degenerative dementia. They found no difference between the groups with respect to the ratio of the two parameters. For both groups the $CMRO_2$/CBF ratio was normal in both the most unaffected and the severely diseased areas. Thus no evidence of chronic hypoxia could be adduced. This important finding suggests that in vascular dementia the brain damage is simply due to sequels after stroke-like acute events just like in the clearcut chronic stroke referred to above. It should be noted that the pathogenesis of the diffuse periventricular white matter changes in Binswanger's disease remains a mystery. It may or may not be the consequence of ischaemia (lack of oxygen).

CBF tomography by SPECT

As CBF and $CMRO_2$ are equally reduced it follows that it suffices to measure CBF in order to obtain an image of the oxygen utilisation that in its turn reflects the brain tissues' functional state. This can be obtained by conventional radio-isotopes using a Rotating Gamma Camera technique, the so-called SPECT procedure (Single Photon Emission Computerised Tomography). SPECT is much less costly than positron camera tomography and technically simpler. It is thus much better suited than PET for routine clinical use.

CBF tomography by SPECT can be recorded by using radioactive Xenon-133, an inert gas administered as inhalation of trace amounts [3,4]. The study lasts only a few minutes and gives quantitative data expressed in milliliters per 100 grams of brain tissue per minute. The study can be repeated after an interval of only 30 min. This means that Xenon-133 can be used for studying the cerebrovascular reserve capacity, comparing the resting state CBF tomograms to those after a vasodilator stimulus such as Diamox (acetazolamide) or carbon dioxide inhalation [5,6].

Technetium-99m is a radioactive isotope which is ideally suited for SPECT. The recent development of Tc-99m labelled compounds as Tc-99m-d,l-HMPAO [7] represents a major technological breakthrough. This tracer is lipophilic and crosses freely into the brain where it is converted to a hydrophilic form that cannot diffuse back to the blood stream. Therefore, the radioactivity is retained in its initial blood flow dominated pattern. The SPECT study lasts about 30 min and permits calculation of CBF in relative units as percentage of CBF in a reference region such as the cerebellum [8]. The validity of the technique has been demonstrated by several comparisons to other well established methods [9–11].

CBF by SPECT in diagnosis of vascular dementia

As mentioned in the introduction it is often difficult to distinguish between vascular and degenerative dementia. The clinical data pointing to cerebrovascular disease as expressed in the Hachinski index [12,13] are not very reliable. Neuroimaging, in particular MRI, is a valuable adjunct, since even chronic infarcts of a fairly small size (lacunes) can be visualised. We, and several other groups, now also use CBF by SPECT for the differential diagnosis. The results so far obtained can be summarised:

1. In vascular dementia the abnormalities noted are in many cases quite mild, corresponding to the cortical and central atrophy often seen on MRI/CT: The blood flow level of the cortex (relative to that of the cerebellum) is reduced and the subcortical region corresponding to the white matter and the lateral ventricles is wider than normal. A most conspicuous absence of the cortical pareito-temporal low flow pattern seen in many patients with degenerative dementia of Alzheimer's type or of marked symmetrical frontal lobe flow reduction seen in other degenerative dementias should also be noted.
2. Moderate and ill demarkated asymmetries of cortical CBF are often found in patients with multiple subcortical lacunar infarcts. These asymmetries probably correspond to disconnection (diaschisis) of the cortex. But the correlation between lacunar infarcts and CBF alterations is not a close one as many such infarcts do not affect CBF measurably. On the other hand, in our series of 10 cases of vascular dementia, of the 4 patients who only had lacunar infarcts, all 4 had such asymmetries. This suggests that in order for subcortical lesions to cause dementia the cortical disconnection must be fairly massive and, it appears, often happens to be asymmetric.
3. In demented patients who have chronic cortical infarcts, the infarcts are sometimes better seen on CBF tomography than on MRI/CT, which tends to show a more diffuse cortical atrophy rendering the recognition of the superimposed focal lesion difficult. The CBF abnormality in a chronic infarct may be fairly sharply demarkated and it often extends far beyond the MRI/CT lesion.
4. The Diamox (acetazolamide) test for measuring the cerebrovascular reserve capacity is negative in most cases of vascular dementia. This is so in patients with multiple lacunar infarcts as well as in patients with chronic cortical infarcts. In the latter case the negative result suggests spontaneous lysis of the arterial thromboembolic occlusion that must have been present when the infarct arose. When positive, as in one of our personal series of patients, the Diamox test indicates vascular occlusion with poor collaterals.

Discussion

Pathoanatomically a vascular aetiology of many dementia cases can be proven or suggested with reasonable certainty. But it has been notoriously difficult to diagnose such cases in vivo. Modern neuroimaging techniques, MRI in particular, are changing this picture, as many parenchymatous lesions of certain presumed vascular aetiology can now be visualised.

In this study we have reviewed the diagnostic value of also recording CBF and $CMRO_2$ tomographically using radioisotopes. This allows one to map the key aetiological factor, the oxygen supply. It could be expected, therefore, that these techniques would be of decisive value in distinguishing vascular dementia from the degenerative dementias such as Alzheimer's disease. This is not so, first of all because ischaemia is not present in the chronic phase when the vascular cases are studied. What is found is a parallel reduction of flow and metabolism in both degenerative and vascular dementia.

Nevertheless, CBF measured by SPECT gave some additional support to the diagnosis. For one thing none of our vascular dementia cases diagnosed clinically and by MRI showed a CBF distribution typical of Alzheimer's disease in milder form, i.e., a reduced CBF in the parieto-temporal regions in both hemispheres. In our Binswanger cases we saw a widening of the subcortical low flow region, and an asymmetry of CBF to the cortex reflecting the impact (diaschisis) caused by the deeper situated lesions.

SPECT was of particular value in defining areas of chronic sequels after cortical infarction. All six patients with such infarcts were very clearly seen on SPECT. This facilitated the interpretation of the MRI abnormalities.

Were there no surprises? We think there were. It surprised us that no less than four out of the ten patients (from the total population of 40 demented and dementia-suspected patients), only one had a very large infarct mainly localised in the cortex. Clinically, the acute phase must have been so 'silent' as to go unnoticed. The mild to moderate dementia in these cases was progressive just like in the Binswanger cases or in the primary degenerative cases of Alzheimer type. It is clear, however, that progressions can be difficult to evaluate on the basis of the anamnestic data alone. And this is usually the clinically relevant situation, even though longitudinal studies are preferable.

These four Single-Infarct-Dementia cases and also our four Binswanger cases suggest to us that the term Multi-Infarct-Dementia is not precise when used to encompass all forms of vascular dementia.

The quest for better in vivo differential diagnosis in dementia is not merely academic in the sense of classifying the diseases and studying their epidemiology. In view of the severity of these disorders for the patients and for society as such, the vascular dementias are of particular interest, as current therapeutics may prevent them or at least arrest their progression.

References

1. Lassen NA, Munck O and Tottey ER (1957) Arch. Neur. Psychiat. 77: 126.
2. Frackowiak RSJ, Pozzilli C, Legg NJ, DuBoulay GM, Marshall J, Lenzi GL and Jones T (1981) Brain 104: 753–778.
3. Stokely EM, Sveinsdottir E, Lassen NA and Rommer P (1980) J. Comput. Assist. Tom. 4: 230–240.
4. Celsis P, Goldman T, Henriksen L and Lassen NA (1981) J. Comput. Assist. Tom. 5: 641–645.
5. Vorstrup S, Engell HC, Lindewald H and Lassen NA (1984) J. Neurosurg. 60: 1070–1075.
6. Vorstrup S, Boysen G, Brun B and Engell NC (1987) Neurol. Res. 9: 10–18.
7. Nowotnik DP, Canning LR, Cumming SA, Harrison RC, Higley B, Nechvatal G et al. (1985) Nucl. Med. Commun. 6: 499–506.

8. Lassen NA, Andersen AR, Friberg L and Paulson OB (1988) J. Cereb. Blood Flow Metab. 8 (suppl. 1): S13–S22.
9. Inugami A, Kanno I, Uemura K, Shishido F, Murakami M, Tomura N, Fujita H and Higano S (1988) J. Cereb. Blood Flow Metab. 8 (suppl. 1): S52–S60.
10. Andersen AR, Friberg H, Schmidt JF and Hasselbalch SG (1988) J. Cereb. Blood Flow Metab. 8 (suppl. 1): S69–S81.
11. Yonekura Y, Nishizawa S, Mukai T, Fujita T, Fukuyama H, Ishikawa M, Kikuchi H, Konishi J, Lassen NA and Andersen AR (1988) J. Cereb. Blood Flow Metab. 8 (suppl. 1): S82–S89.
12. Hachinski VC, Iliff LD, Zilkha E, DuBoulay GH, McAllister VL, Marshall J, Ross Russell RW and Symon L (1975) Arch. Neurol. (Chicago) 32: 632–637.
13. Harrison MJG, Thomas DJ, DuBoulay GH and Marshall J (1979) J. Neurol. Sci. 40: 97–103.

Vascular disease and dementia

Michael D. O'Brien
Department of Neurology, Guy's Hospital, St Thomas' Street, London SE1 9RT, UK

Introduction

The role of cerebrovascular disease in the development of dementia has been a matter of controversy in recent years [1,2]. This paper will consider only two aspects; firstly, how important is cerebrovascular disease as a cause of dementia, and secondly, how does cerebrovascular disease cause dementia.

Table 1 shows the wide variety of vascular diseases that may be associated with dementia and emphasises the point that vascular dementia is not a homogeneous disease entity, but may be the consequence of any disturbance of blood supply to the brain from any cause.

The importance of cerebrovascular disease as a cause of dementia

Much of the controversy is due to confusion about the definition of vascular dementia. Many of the conditions listed in Table 1 cause large discrete infarcts. Most of these patients suffer from some loss of intellectual function, even if this deficit is quite circumscribed, or could only be demonstrated on special psychological tests. These patients are not usually included with patients described as having a vascular dementia, nor is it useful to do so. There is a spectrum which ranges from these patients with stroke at one end, to those who have a vascular cause of dementia which is clinically indistinguishable from Alzheimer's disease at the other end. Most published series on vascular dementia have opted to include patients whose main or presenting feature was dementia and in whom subsequent evaluation has shown a vascular cause. However, this division is clearly arbitrary and the point at which patients are diagnosed as having a vascular dementia, and not some intellectual impairment associated with an evident stroke, has not been determined. This issue alone would result in very large differences in the estimates of prevalence of vascular dementia.

This problem of definition needs to be resolved before the relative contribution of vascular disease can be determined and even then there are major difficulties deciding whether vascular disease is the cause of the dementia, contributes to it, or is purely coincidental.

Table 1. Vascular causes of dementia

1. Due to or associated with hypertension
   a) Binswanger's disease
   b) Small vessel arteriosclerosis
   c) Lacunar state
   d) Hypertensive encephalopathy
2. Cardiac disease
   a) Embolic.
   b) Hypoperfusion leading to watershed infarcts
3. Arteriosclerosis (large vessel disease)
   a) Embolic
   b) Low flow
4. Amyloid angiopathy
   a) Sporadic
   b) Familial
5. Cerebral vasculitis
   a) Primary
   b) Associated with a systemic vasculitis
6. Postural hypotension (Shy-Drager or multi-system atrophy)
7. Polycythaemia
8. Granular cortical atrophy (cortical micro-infarcts)

Some research protocols have required the selection of patients in whom the dementia is unequivocally of vascular origin and this has been done on clinical criteria, which is the basis of the ischaemia score formulated by Hachinski et al. [3], and by CT scan or MRI appearances. The ischaemia score has been widely used to identify these patients and it is based on the different presentation and clinical course of Alzheimer's disease and vascular disease, weighting factors which are thought to be more typical of a stroke-like illness compared to the insidious development of dementia in Alzheimer's disease. Hachinski [4] has said that the ischaemia score is designed to identify strokes, which of course it does, but only large or clinically evident strokes, everything else is necessarily included in the Alzheimer group. The score therefore does not divide patients into a vascular group and an Alzheimer group, but rather into an eloquent infarct group and everything else; into the 'everything else' group go those patients with vascular dementia but without clinically evident strokes and most of the mixed cases. This also applies the other way, for example, a patient with Alzheimer's disease who has a stroke early in the course of the disease, perhaps even before the dementia is very obvious, will be classified in the multi-infarct group.

Patients who definitely have a vascular cause can be identified with up to an 85% accuracy and may therefore satisfy the criteria for inclusion in a particular study, such as measurements of cerebral blood flow or metabolism or assessment of risk factors, but these methods of selection would not detect all those with a vascular aetiology or significant vascular contribution from an unselected group of demented patients. This is evident from the fact that these methods only identify a vascular cause for dementia in 10–15% of patients, whereas pathological studies indicate that the figure is more like 30–40%.

Pathological studies might be expected to resolve some of these difficulties, but they can only quantify the amount of abnormality and its distribution, they cannot say anything about the function of the brain and an additional problem is that pathological studies necessarily represent the end stage of the disease process and do not identify the amount or distribution of pathological abnormalities in the very early stages of the disease, at a time when intervention might have some effect on prognosis [5].

In most of the published series there has been little difficulty in identifying patients with Alzheimer's disease and those with just vascular disease, particularly in younger patients. None of the published series had shown any success in identifying patients with both diseases and, of course, this is likely to be the situation in a large number of elderly patients. Even if both diseases could be identified it would still be extremely difficult to determine whether the dementia was due to the presence of two diseases together, or whether one disease was the cause of the dementia and the other co-incidental.

Table 2 shows the percentages of Alzheimer's disease, vascular disease and mixed cases in a number of published papers. The pure vascular group range from 9–59%, the mixed Alzheimer and vascular group range from 4–23%, giving a total vascular contribution of 13–63%.

Only the papers by Tomlinson et al. [6] and Ulrich et al. [8], express some uncertainty about how confident they could be in ascribing the dementia to a particular pathological process; in this context it is of some interest that all the other series had no such difficulty. Tomlinson [7] found that 50% of their patients had significant Alzheimer's disease and no greater volume of infarction than was found in the control group. They divided the vascular group into 'definite' and 'probable'. The definite vascular group, amounting to 12%, were those with volumes of softening in excess of 100 ml and none of his control subjects exceeded this volume. These patients had no significant Alzheimer's disease. This left four

Table 2. Percentages of Alzheimer's disease, vascular disease and mixed cases in the literature

	Ref. no.	No. of pts.	% Alzheimer	% Mixed	% Vascular	% Total vascular
Tomlinson et al. (1970)	6	50	50	8–18	12–18	20–36
Ulrich et al. (1982)	8	54	37–57	11–19	17–20	28–39
Malamud (1972)	10	1225	42	23	29	52
Molsa et al. (1985)	11	58	48	10	19	29
Esiri & Wilcock (1986)	12	86	40	13	21	33
Barclay et al. (1985)	13	311	64	14	22	36
Wade et al. (1987)	15	65	58	15	9	24
Homer et al. (1988)	14	27	22	4	59	63
Boller et al. (1989)	16	54	68	4	9	13

patients (8%) with volumes of cerebral softening of about 100 ml associated with a moderate or large amount of Alzheimer's disease, and it is likely that both pathological processes were contributory.

Ulrich et al. [8] found some of the changes associated with Alzheimer's disease in 53 out of their 54 patients (98%), but using the same criteria as Tomlinson, 57% were thought to have significant Alzheimer pathology. The undoubted vascular dementias ranged from 17–20% according to criteria used, but Ulrich et al. chose a different method of dividing the mixed cases. They found one group of 11% in whom there was sufficient vascular disease and Alzheimer pathology for both diseases alone to have caused the dementia. The other mixed group were those in whom the dementia was thought to have been caused by the combination of the two diseases and this group ranged from 0–8%, according to the criteria used. From this series therefore, the vascular contribution to dementia ranged from a minimum of 28% to a maximum of 39%.

How does cerebrovascular disease cause dementia?

One of the problems is that not all patients with cerebral vascular disease are demented, so why is it that some develop dementia and others do not? Is it a matter of the volume of infarcted brain? What about the effects of bilateral lesions? Can strategically placed small lesions cause dementia? What is the underlying pathological process in Binswanger's disease, leukoariosis and granular cortical atrophy? Is it all a matter of infarcts, large and small, or do these patients have a significant population of ischaemia but viable cells? Is treatment only to be directed at preventing further ischaemia episodes or is it possible to produce some improvement in cells already ischaemic?

All the pathological studies summarised in Table 2 are based on the volume of infarction, but the problem is not why is the patient with 300–400 ml of cerebral softening demented, but rather why is the patient with only small volumes of infarction demented. Erkinjuntti et al. [7] have recently reported a series of neuropathologically verified cases of vascular dementia. The mean volume of infarction was only 40 ml, but the range was 1–229 ml and of course, it should be reemphasised that pathological studies are necessarily the end stage of the pathological process. It seems clear therefore that there is a very wide variation between patients, some with quite large volumes of infarction may not be demented and patients with quite small infarcts may be demented, and there were five patients in Erkinjuntti's series with 1 ml or less of infarcted tissue; so we must conclude that the development of dementia is not just related to the volume of infarction.

Pathological studies have also emphasised the importance of bilateral lesions. In Tomlinson's series bilateral lesions was a striking feature in his vascular group and 96% of Erkinjuntti's patients had bilateral lesions, so it seems that bilateral lesions may be more significant than a single lesion whose volume is greater than the two lesions combined. To this we have to add the location of lesions. In Tomlinson's series, infarction of the hippocampus and adjacent limbic structures was found in 14% of patients with dementia and in none of the control group and infarction of the corpus callosum was only found in patients with dementia. In Erkinjuntti's series, temporal lobes were involved in 91% and the basal ganglia in 83%.

Lesions affecting the deep white matter particularly of the frontal lobes, as in Binswanger's disease and etat lacunar, are more likely to be significant because of their bilaterality and location than the volume of affected tissue.

An unsolved question is whether in these patients there is a significant number of ischaemic but viable cells and this is clearly a matter of considerable importance with regard to possible treatment. Early cerebral blood flow studies using the Rety-Schmidt technique showed an increased arteriovenous oxygen difference in some patients with dementia, implying a greater extraction of oxygen due to an inadequate blood supply [5]. However, PET studies have not shown convincing evidence that neurones are viable but ischaemic, and oxygen extraction ratios for both oxygen and glucose have been virtually normal. However, we know that the potential for this situation exists from the experimental cerebral blood flow work showing a gap of about 10 ml/100 g/min between loss of function and complete infarction and furthermore, that the cells in this state are potentially retrievable.

The prospective study of Rogers et al. [18] has shown that patients who develop a vascular dementia may have profoundly reduced cerebral blood flow for some years before there is any clinical evidence of dementia, whereas in patients with Alzheimer's disease the onset of dementia is associated with a reduction in flow which then parallels the progression of the disease. These authors have also shown that attention to the risk factors for vascular disease improves the prognosis; a finding which suggests that there is a process of ischaemia which starts some years before the development of dementia in patients some of which might be retrievable.

Conclusion

The evidence suggests that vascular disease is the second most common cause of dementia and that at least one third of all patients dying with dementia have a significant vascular component. Cerebrovascular disease causes dementia by a combination of the volume of infarcted tissue, the location of the lesions and particularly their bilaterality and all three of these factors are important. The volume of infarcted tissue alone is not an adequate indication of dementia. Ischaemia without infarction certainly exists, but whether this persists sufficiently long and affects a sufficient number of cells to be clinically significant remains undetermined.

References

1. O'Brien MD (1988) Vascular dementia is underdiagnosed. Arch. Neurol. 45: 797–798.

2. Brust JCM (1988) Vascular dementia is overdiagnosed. Arch. Neurol. 45: 799–801.
3. Hachinski VC, Iliff LD, Zilkha E, du Boulay GH, McAllister VL, Marshall J, Ross Russell RW and Symon L (1975) Cerebral blood flow and dementia. Arch. Neurol. 32: 632–637.
4. Hachinski VC (1983) Multifocal dementia. Neuro. Clin. 1: 27–36.
5. O'Brien MD (1977) Vascular disease and dementia in the elderly. In: Lynn Smith W and Kinsbourne M (eds.) Aging and Dementia. Spectrum, New York, pp. 77–90.
6. Tomlinson BE, Blessed S and Roth M (1970) Observations on the brain of demented old people. J. Neurol. Sci. 11: 205–242.
7. Tomlinson BE (1977) Morphological change and dementia in old age. In: Lynn Smith W and Kinsbourne M (eds.) Aging and Dementia. Spectrum, New York, pp. 25–56.
8. Ulrich J, Probst A and Wuest M (1986) The brain diseases causing senile dementia. J. Neurol. 233: 118–722.
9. Erkinjuntti T, Maltia M, Palo J, Sulkava R and Paetau A (1988) Accuracy of the clinical diagnosis of vascular dementia: A prospective clinical and postmortem neuropathological study. J. Neurol. Neurosurg. Psychiat. 51: 1037–1044.
10. Malamud N (1972) Neuropathology of organic brain syndromes associated with aging. In: Gaitz CM (ed.) Aging and the Brain. Plenum, New York 14: 497–506.
11. Molsa PK, Paljarvi L, Rinne JD, Rinne UK and Sako E (1985) Validity of clinical diagnosis in dementia: A prospective clinicopathological study. J. Neurol. Neurosurg. Psychiat. 48: 1085–1090.
12. Esiri M and Wilcock GK (1986) Cerebral amyloid angiopathy in dementia and old age. J. Neurol. Neurosurg. Psychiat. 49: 1221–1226.
13. Barclay L, Zemcov A, Blass JP and Sansone J (1985) Survival in Alzheimer's disease and vascular dementias. Neurology 35: 834–840.
14. Homer AC, Honavar M, Lantos PL, Hastie IR, Kellett JM and Millard PH (1988) Diagnosing dementia: Do we get it right. Br. Med. J. 297: 894–896.
15. Wade JPH, Mirgen TR, Hachinski VC, Fishman M, Lau C and Merskey H (1987) The clinical diagnosis of Alzheimer disease. Arch. Neurol. 44: 24–29.
16. Boller F, Lopez O and Moossy J (1989) Diagnosis of dementia: Clinicopathological correlations. Neurology 38: 76–79.
17. Erkinjuntti T, Haltia M, Palo J, Sulkava R and Paetau A (1988) Accuracy of the clinical diagnosis of vascular dementia. J. Neuro. Neurosurg. Psychiat. 51: 1037–1044.
18. Rogers RL, Meyer JS, Mortel KF and Mahurin RK (1986) Decreased cerebral blood flow precedes multi-infarct dementia, but follows senile dementia of the Alzheimer type. Neurology 36: 1–6.

The assessment of multi-infarct dementia

Vladimir Hachinski
Department of Clinical Neurological Sciences, University of Western Ontario and the John P. Robarts Research Institute, University Hospital, P.O. Box 5339, London, Ontario N6A 5A5, Canada

Introduction

The assessment of multi-infarct dementia (MID) remains difficult because it attempts to identify an entity that commonly coexists and interacts with Alzheimer's disease. Nevertheless, a systematic, stepwise approach usually yields the correct diagnosis or at least the identification of vascular factors in the dementia under consideration.

Clinical assessment

Clinical assessment remains the mainstay and most reliable method of assessing multi-infarct dementia. It involves three overlapping steps.

Determining dementia

The clinical *history* obtained through the patient, relatives, co-workers and friends can best document the development of a persistent impairment of intellectual function. The *physical examination* may reveal the presence of primitive reflexes, suggesting a chronic, diffuse process; focal neurological findings or signs characteristic of specific neurological syndromes such as Parkinson's disease. The degree and type of mental deterioration can be determined by bedside *mental status scales* such as the Mini-Mental State [1,2] or the Blessed Score [3]. Whenever possible, formal standardized *psychometrics* are desirable both for assessing severity and as a baseline to document progression, stability or improvement.

The clinical assessment is also most likely to yield clues about conditions masquerading as dementia such as depression, focal neurological syndromes and drug intoxication.

Determining the type of dementia

Huntington's disease, Parkinsonism, normal pressure hydrocephalus, Pick's dis-

Table 1. Ischemic score

Abrupt onset	2
Stepwise deterioration	1
Fluctuating course	2
Nocturnal confusion	1
Relative preservation of personality	1
Depression	1
Somatic complaints	1
Emotional incontinence	1
History of hypertension	1
History of strokes	2
Evidence of associated atherosclerosis	1
Focal neurological symptoms	2
Focal neurological signs	2

A score of 4 or less suggests a diagnosis of Alzheimer's disease. A score of 7 or more suggests a diagnosis of MID.

ease, and several other syndromes have characteristic clinical presentations. The clinical evaluation will also uncover the need to rule out other conditions such as hypothyroidism, vitamin B12 deficiency, brain tumor, subdural hematomas, and other rare causes of dementia.

Distinguishing between Alzheimer's disease and MID

This constitutes the most common clinical situation. Despite well founded criticisms, particularly those of Liston and LaRue [4], the ischemic score [5] remains the single most useful method of distinguishing between the two entities (Table 1).

A difficulty with the ischemic score is that the items were not well defined. This shortcoming has been partially redressed [6,7].

Abrupt onset refers to the onset of intellectual decline, not to be confused with sudden recognition. Patients may cope in a familiar setting despite considerable intellectual decline. Intercurrent illness or the death of a spouse can precipitate a crisis, falsely suggesting an acute onset. *Stepwise deterioration* characterizes plateaus of stable cognition interrupted by episodes of rapid deterioration. A *fluctuating course* implies a temporal profile of improvement from one cerebral infarct followed by decline from the next.

Nocturnal confusion implies relative daytime lucidity since nocturnal exacerbations are a feature common to all types of dementia. Episodes of nocturnal wandering are considered more characteristic of vascular dementia than Alzheimer's disease [8]. Insight and emotional responsiveness tend to be preserved for longer in patients with MID than Alzheimer's disease, and hence the item of *relative preservation of personality*. Perhaps as a consequence, depressive symptomatology is found more frequently in MID than Alzheimer's disease. *Somatic complaints* refer to vague and usually inexplicable symptoms such as dizziness, unsteadiness or headache of which patients with MID often complain. Sometimes these undoubtedly reflect an underlying affective disorder; on other occasions an organic basis is suspected. Whatever their etiology, this should be scored whenever non-specific symptoms without obvious physical counterparts are prominent.

Emotional incontinence refers to the rapid, exaggerated, and inappropriate swings in emotional manifestations often seen in patients with bilateral cortico-bulbar lesions. It can be prominent in the lacunar state, and by contrast, is most unusual in Alzheimer's disease.

A *history of hypertension* and/or its confirmation on examination favor a diagnosis of MID, since hypertension is a major risk factor for all types of stroke. The incidence of stroke is higher in patients with a history of associated *atherosclerosis* (ischemic heart disease, intermittent claudication), and even when the history is negative, the finding of a carotid bruit or absent foot pulses would lend support to a vascular etiology. A *history of strokes* certainly suggests MID but in itself is insufficient to make the diagnosis, since patients with Alzheimer's disease may also suffer from stroke.

Focal neurological symptoms include visual disturbances, brain stem abnormalities (such as dysarthria, dysphagia and ataxia) and episodes of sensory disturbance or weakness in the limbs. Symptoms may be transient, suggesting a TIA, or persist, as in completed stroke. Dysphasia, dyscalculia, dyspraxia, agnosia and other symptoms which may be due to focal cortical lesions are excluded simply because they have little discriminant value, since they are common to both Alzheimer's disease and MID. The same considerations apply to neurological signs, and again the score achieves greater discrimination if we exclude signs attributable to cortical lesions. The exception is a homonymous hemianopia, which may be due to an occipital cortical lesion, since this is rarely, if ever, seen in Alzheimer's disease. Accordingly any visual-field defect of central origin is included as a focal sign.

Primitive reflexes are common to both groups and are therefore excluded unless they are clearly asymmetrical. Signs of brain-stem dysfunction (cranial nerve palsy, pseudobulbar palsy) are scored as focal signs. In the limbs, any evidence of cortico-spinal involvement, including an isolated Babinski sign, is taken as a focal sign, since long tract signs are extremely uncommon in Alzheimer's disease [9]. Discretion must be exercised regarding coincidental peripheral neuropathies, root lesions, and other unrelated focal signs unlikely to help in the differentiation of MID from Alzheimer's disease. A focal neurological sensory sign refers to a loss of sensation of central but non-cortical nature. Thus hemisensory loss to pain and temperature perception would be acceptable, but not astereognosis or graphesthesia.

In addition to Rosen et al.'s [10] clinico-pathological validation of some of the items of the ischemic score, Cummings et al. [11] have confirmed that depression is significantly more common in MID than in Alzheimer's disease. The fact that sleep apnea occurs more commonly in MID than in Alzheimer's disease [12] supports nocturnal confusion as a valid criterion. Meyer et al. [13] showed that intellectual function fluctuated in patients with MID whereas it showed a steady decline in patients with Alzheimer's disease, justifying fluctuating course as an item in the ischemic score. Despite the above evidence the ischemic score needs further definition, refinement, and validation.

Clinico-pathological studies coincide in finding the ischemic score reliable in distinguishing MID from Alzheimer's disease but unable to discriminate between MID and mixed dementia [10,14,15]. Perhaps this is to be expected, given the common occurrence of Alzheimer's disease and cerebral infarction with increasing age. From a practical standpoint it may not matter much, since it is the identification of a vascular component that is potentially subject to treatment and prevention.

Radiological assessment

Computerized tomography (CT) of the brain marked a major advance in diagnosis. CT can rule out mass lesions, suggest communicating hydrocephalus, document atrophy, and identify infarcts; but it cannot make the diagnosis of MID. Although the presence of infarcts on CT correlates with the diagnosis of MID, inclusion of CT criteria does not increase the accuracy of the ischemic score [14]. Perhaps this should not be surprising. A patient may suffer several major cerebral infarcts without becoming demented and conversely a small strategically placed lesion, such as an infarct in the left anterior thalamus, may devastate cognition. CT infarcts have to be related to the clinical picture in terms of their size, site, recency and the presence of other lesions or pathological processes.

The CT also identifies leukoaraiosis [16] which occurred in 33% of Alzheimer's disease patients and in all cases of MID in one CT studied series [17] Erkinjuntti et al. [14] found that white matter low attenuation differentiated MID and probable vascular dementia patients from Alzheimer patients. However, many controversies remain regarding the interpretation of white matter changes and their significance [18].

Magnetic resonance imagining (MRI) has all the advantages of CT scanning and a great potential for advancing the assessment of MID. However, at the moment MRI shows us much more than we can interpret.

Neurophysiological assessment

Electroencephalography (EEG) distinguishes patients with Alzheimer's and mixed dementia from aged matched control subjects, and in individuals coming to autopsy quantified neuronal loss correlates with the severity of the EEG abnormalities [19]. Although focal EEG abnormalities are more common in MID than in Alzheimer's disease [20,21], the findings are not specific enough for diagnosing individual patients.

Short latency somatosensory evoked potentials tends to be normal in patients with Alzheimer's disease whereas patients with MID show a prolongation of central conduction time, longer latencies for the N13 and N20 components and diminished primary cortical response amplitude [22]. This is an intriguing observation that deserves confirmation.

Cerebral blood flow and metabolism

Cerebral blood flow (CBF) measurements are not a reliable measure of ischemia, because a low CBF may simply reflect a low metabolic demand and not ischemia. Positron emission tomography (PET) studies do provide a means of measuring CBF and metabolism simultaneously and thus assessing the possibility of ischemia. Frackowiak et al. [23] in a study of 9 MID and 13 degenerative dementia patients concluded that both groups had general and focal decreases of CBF and metabolism and that these were coupled, i.e., there was no disparity between CBF and metabolism as would be expected in a state of chronic ischemia. PET scanning is a powerful technique for elucidating the pathophysiology of vascular dementia but its findings are not yet applicable to daily practice.

Conclusion

The assessment of MID remains preeminently clinical. Despite limitations, the ischemic score remains an easy, inexpensive, and valid method of diagnosing MID. Identification of infarcts in images of the brain must be interpreted in accordance with the clinical picture, and the management should be guided by the specific etiology causing these infarcts.

Acknowledgements

Dr Hachinski is a Career Investigator of the Heart and Stroke Foundation of Ontario.

References

1. Folstein MF, Folstein SE and McHugh PR (1975) 'Mini-Mental State,' A practical method for grading the cognitive state of patients for the clinician. J. Psychiat. Res. 12: 189–198.
2. Anthony JC, LeResche L, Niaz U, von Korff MR and Folstein MF (1982) Limits of the 'Mini-Mental State' as a screening test for dementia and delirium among hospital patients. Psychol. Med. 12: 397–408.
3. Blessed G, Tomlinson BE and Roth M (1968) The association between quantitative measures of dementia and of senile change in the cerebral grey matter of elderly subjects. Appendix, Br. J. Psychiat. 114: 797–811.

4. Liston EH and LaRue A (1983) Clinical differentiation of primary degenerative and multi-infarct dementia: A critical review of the evidence. Part II: Pathological studies. Bio Psychiat. 18: 1467–1483.
5. Hachinski VC, Iliff LD, Phil M et al. (1975) Cerebral blood flow in dementia. Arch. Neurol. 32: 632–637.
6. Hachinski VC (1983) Multi-infarct dementia. Neurol. Clin. 1: 27–36.
7. Wade JPH and Hachinski VC (1987) Multi-infarct dementia. In: Pitt BM (ed.) Dementia (Medicine in Old Age). Churchill Livingstone, London, England, pp. 209–228.
8. Roth M (1981) The diagnosis of dementia in late and middle life. In: Mortimer JA and Shuman LM (eds.). The Epidemiology of Dementia. Oxford University Press, New York, pp. 31–33.
9. Koller WC, Wilson RS, Glatt SL and Fox JH (1984) Motor signs are infrequent in dementia of the Alzheimer type. Ann. Neurol. 16: 514–516.
10. Rosen WG, Terry RD, Fuld PA, Katzman R and Peck A (1979) Pathologic verification of ischemic score in differentiation of dementia. Ann. Neurol. 7: 486–488.
11. Cummings JL, Miller B, Hill MA and Neshkes R (1987) Neuropsychiatric aspects of multi-infarct dementia and dementia of the Alzheimer type. Arch. Neurol. 44: 389–393.
12. Erkinjuntti T, Partinen M, Sulkava R, Telakivi T, Salmi T and Tilvis R (1987) Sleep apnea in multi-infarct dementia and Alzheimer's disease. Sleep 10: 419–425.
13. Meyer JS, Rogers RL, Judd BW, Mortel KF and Sims P (1988) Cognition and cerebral blood flow fluctuate together in multi-infarct dementia. Stroke 19: 163–169.
14. Erkinjuntti T (1987) Differential diagnosis between Alzheimer's disease and vascular dementia: Evaluation of common clinical methods. Acta Neurol. Scand. 76: 433–442.
15. Wade JPH, Mirsen TR, Hachinski VC, Fisman M, Lau C and Merskey H (1987) The clinical diagnosis of Alzheimer's disease. Arch. Neurol. 44: 24–29.
16. Hachinski VC, Potter P and Merskey H (1987) Leukoaraiosis. Arch. Neurol. 44: 21–23.
17. Inzitari D, Diaz JF, Fox AJ et al. (1987) Vascular risk factors and leukoaraiosis. Arch. Neurol. 44: 42–47.
18. Brown MM and Hachinski VC (1989) Vascular dementia. In: Current Opinion in Neurology and Neurosurgery vol. 2, pp. 78–84.
19. Rae-Grant AD, Blume WT, Lau C, Hachinski VC, Fisman M and Merskey H (1987) The electroencephalogram in Alzheimer type dementia: A sequential study correlating the electroencephalogram with psychometric and quantitative pathological data. Arch. Neurol. 44: 50–54.
20. Roberts MA, McGeorge AP and Laird FI (1978) Electroencephalography and computerized tomography in vascular and non-vascular dementia in old age. J. Neurol. Neurosurg. Psychiatry 41: 903–906.
21. Harrison MJG, Thomas DJ, Du Boulay GH, Marshall J: Multi infarct dementia. J. Neurol. Sci. 40: 97–103.
22. Abbruzzese G, Reni L, Cocito L et al. (1984) Short latency somatosensory evoked potentials in degenerative and vascular dementia. J. Neurol. Neurosurg. Psychiatry 47: 1034–1037.
23. Frackowiak RSJ, Pozzilli C, Legg NJ et al. (1981) Regional cerebral oxygen supply and utilization in dementia. Brain 104: 753–778.

The design of clinical trials on vascular dementia

Ronald S. Black and John P. Blass
Dementia Research Service, Cornell University Medical College at the Burke Rehabilitation Center, White Plains, NY 10605, USA

Damage to the brain from vascular disease is, after Alzheimer disease, the second most common cause of the dementia syndrome. Longitudinal studies have demonstrated that approximately 10–20% of patients with the dementia syndrome have vascular dementia; an approximately equal percentage have 'mixed dementia' in which degenerative and vascular causes both contribute to the cognitive impairment [1,2]. The design of therapeutic trials for vascular dementia is complicated by the heterogeneous nature of the disorder [3]. At least four syndromes of cognitive impairment result from abnormalities in the supply of blood and oxygen to the brain. One is brain damage secondary to an episode of generalized hypoxia (e.g., carbon monoxide poisoning) and/or ischemia (e.g., cardiac arrest) [4]. A second is the cognitive deficits which can accompany the motor and sensory sequelae of major strokes. A third syndrome is progressive dementia attributable to multiple small infarcts [5]. In such patients, focal neurologic signs attributable to specific episodes of minor stroke typically accompany the dementia; imaging studies will demonstrate discrete areas of infarction in the cerebral hemispheres. Despite the common use of the term 'multi-infarct dementia' for all forms of vascular dementia, this form of dementia appears to be quite rare; it accounted for only 3 of 200 consecutive patients in the dementia clinic of Larson et al. [6].

The fourth group of patients consists of those with the dementia syndrome as a consequence of diffuse damage to the white matter of the cerebral hemispheres. Otto Binswanger first emphasized the potential role of vascular damage to the white matter as a cause of progressive dementia in 1894 [7]; since that time the nature and even the existence of Binswanger disease have been the subject of controversy [8,9]. Caplan and Schoene [8] concluded that Binswanger encephalopathy in its 'pure form' represents one of the 'extremes of a clinical spectrum'. Patients with such diffuse white matter damage are clinically heterogenous; they may develop significant abnormalities of motor function, such as gait disturbances, or may be clinically indistinguishable from patients with Alzheimer disease [8–10]. Typical pathological findings include loss of myelin, gliosis, hyalinization of arterioles, atherosclerosis including smaller arteries, and small lacunar infarcts [10]. Recent electron microscopic studies suggest capillaries may be involved as well [11]. Numerous etiologies have been proposed for this disorder, all involving compromise of the circulation, including atherosclerosis [12], thickening and hyalinization of arterioles [13], venous thrombosis [14,15], hydrocephalus [9,16], chronic edema [17,18], hypertension [8,9], and hypoperfusion [8,18]. The sensitivity of white matter to circulatory impairments agrees with experimental data. In physiologically stabilized animals subjected to controlled mild hypoxia, metabolic changes were much more marked in white matter than in gray, perhaps because the vascular tree in white matter is less lush [19].

Imaging studies are less useful in the diagnosis of this condition. Computerized tomography may show patchy or diffuse areas of decreased attenuation in the hemispheric white matter – termed leukoaraiosis by Hachinski et al. [20]. Studies have found, however, that this finding may be a non-specific accompaniment of normal aging [21,22]. Steingart et al. [23] studied 105 'normal' elderly subjects and found 9 with CT evidence of leukoaraiosis [8.6%]. These nine patients, however, were found to have significantly lower scores on psychometric testing and may have had subclinical cognitive impairment. A more significant problem, though more difficult to quantify, is that patients with diffuse damage to the hemispheric white matter may have normal CT scans [24]. Similar problems are encountered in the interpretation of magnetic resonance imaging (MRI) studies. MRI scans may be normal in the presence of cerebral infarction. Kertesz et al. [25] studied 100 patients with clinical stroke and found that 21 had no lesion on MRI scan. A more important limitation in the interpretation of MRI studies is the very high proportion of normal subjects in this elderly population who will have abnormalities on MRI. In this same study [25] a population of age matched control subjects was used, between ages 50 and 78 (mean age 60.5 years). In this group of 58 subjects, only 13 had no lesion on MRI scan (22%). The incidence of abnormalities such as periventricular 'rims' and 'caps' of hyperintensity as well as foci of hyperintensity in the subcortical white matter (commonly called UBOs – unidentified bright objects) was found to increase with age. The severity and number of signal abnormalities were increased in the patients with clinical stroke. However, the percentage of patients with subcortical hyperintensities on MRI scan was similar in the stroke (21%) and normal control (22%) groups. In addition, recent reports of abnormalities of periventricular signal in scans obtained with high field strength magnets (1.5 T) occurring in Alzheimer disease further complicate the interpretation of MRI scans in the diagnosis of dementia [26]. Given the potential for false negatives in the use of CT scans to diagnose vascular dementia and the potential for false positives in the use of MRI, Barclay [27] has calculated that both are of approximately equal value in the diagnosis of vascular dementia. Based on this analysis she suggests that in clinical trials for Alzheimer disease MRI be used to discriminate between vascular and degenerative causes of dementia, while in clinical trials for vascular dementia CT be used to discriminate between these diagnoses.

An alternative approach to the classification of patients with suspected vascular dementia is to rely solely on clinical criteria for diagnosis. The modified ischemia score of Hachinski has been used to identify patients with a high probability of dementia due to vascular causes [28]. This scale combines questions related to the patient's history, clinical course, neurological evaluation, and associated symptoms to produce an 'ischemia score'. A score of six or greater is considered positive. Autopsy studies have shown that this score is a highly useful, although not invariably accurate predictor of vascular disease of the brain [29,30]. The Diagnostic and Statistical Manual of Mental Disorders provides clinical criteria for the diagnosis of vascular dementia (termed multi-infarct dementia) which is not reliant on imaging data [31]. Diagnosis of multi-infarct dementia by these criteria requires the presence of a dementia with a stepwise deteriorating course, focal neurological signs and symptoms, and 'evidence from history, physical examination, or laboratory tests of significant cerebrovascular disease that is judged to be etiologically related to the disturbance.' Thus imaging studies can be used to arrive at this conclusion, but need not be abnormal to make the diagnosis.

These clinical criteria for vascular dementia were used to select patients for a single center, double blind placebo controlled trial of pentoxifylline (Trental) in vascular dementia. Patients who met DSM-III criteria for multi-infarct dementia and had a modified Hachinski score of 6 or more were eligible if they demonstrated a moderate degree of cognitive impairment as defined by Mini-Mental Status Examination [32] score (6–27 out of 30, inclusive) and Alzheimer Disease Assessment Scale (ADAS, 33) score (15–60). Eligible patients were also at least 55 years old, and were generally in good medical health; significant medical conditions had to be stable on medication for at least one month before enrollment. History of major depression and use of psychotropic medication were among the other exclusion criteria.

All patients had either CT or MRI scans before enrollment, however the imaging results were not used as inclusion or exclusion criteria. Sixty-four patients were enrolled between August 1984 and March 1987. Of these 64 patients 48 had CT alone, 2 had MRI alone, and 14 had MRI and CT. Forty-one patients (64%) had infarcts or evidence of white matter damage on either CT or MRI. Of the 62 patients who had CT scans and met these strict clinical criteria for vascular dementia, only 30 (48%) had infarcts or white matter damage demonstrated on CT; of the 16 patients who had MRI scans 15 had these changes (94%). Of the 32 patients without evidence of infarcts or damage to the white matter on CT 15 scans were read as normal and 17 had atrophy out of proportion to the patient's age. A subgroup of 37 patients with a clear-cut clinical history of stroke was defined; 27 (73%) of these patients had infarcts or white matter damage on CT or MRI (10 of 26 CTs and 7 of 7 MRIs were positive). Even in the presence of a clinical history of stroke a substantial percentage of patients with a clinical diagnosis of vascular dementia (which by DSM-III criteria requires focal neurologic signs) had no evidence of infarcts or white matter damage on CT scan. The high percentage of these abnormalities on MRI scans in these patients must be viewed in light of the high percentage of normal elderly subjects with these MRI findings, as discussed above [25]. Positive imaging studies may only define a subgroup of patients with vascular dementia.

This study was defined as a double-blind, parallel group comparison of oral pentoxifylline (400 mg three times daily) vs. placebo. A 36 week duration of treatment was planned. The primary outcome measure was designated a priority as the total score on the ADAS, and the study protocol specified that the result would be considered positive if the rate of deterioration in the total ADAS score for patients receiving pentoxifylline was significantly less than that for patients who received placebo ($P < 0.05$, one tailed test). End point analysis of mean decrease in ADAS total score revealed that patients on pentoxifylline had significantly less deterioration on this measure than patients on placebo ($P = 0.029$). The result was similar when only the cognitive measures from the ADAS (items 1–7) were taken into account; pentoxifylline patients deteriorated less ($P = 0.018$). When mean ADAS score at the beginning of the trial was compared with the mean score at the end of the trial for the patients who completed the trial (36 weeks), there was significant deterioration in the placebo group (11.1 ± 3.01, $p < 0.01$ from baseline, 18 patients) while the patients receiving pentoxifylline deteriorated less (3.10 ± 2.48, not significantly different from baseline, 20 patients). Similarly, the mean endpoint ADAS score for all 32 placebo patients was significantly less than the baseline mean ($P < 0.01$, mean decrease 7.00 ± 2.12) while the mean endpoint ADAS score for all 32 pentoxifylline patients was not significantly different from baseline (mean decrease, 1.70 ± 1.72). Pentoxifylline appears to have a positive effect on the course of vascular dementia as defined in this study, significantly slowing the rate of deterioration in these patients.

These encouraging results demonstrate the possible efficacy of a treatment for this common form of dementia, and agree with the results of less extensive trials in other countries [34,35]. Further studies with larger numbers of patients, in various stages of the disease, and over longer periods of time are needed. The use of imaging studies to define this syndrome is likely to remain an area of controversy. Advances in magnetic resonance imaging technology, such as high field strength imaging will not necessarily improve the accuracy of a diagnosis of vascular dementia, as the number of cognitively intact elderly subjects with white matter abnormalities may increase; further advances in the ability to interpret these abnormalities will also be required.

References

1. Kokmen E, Offord KP and Okasaki H (1987) A clinical and autopsy study of dementia in Olmstead County, Minnesota. Neurology 37: 426–430.
2. Shoenberg BS, Kokmen E and Okasaki H (1987) Alzheimer's disease and other dementing illnesses in a defined United States population: Incidence rates and clinical features. Ann. Neurol. 22: 724–729.
3. Blass JP (1987) Circulatory and degenerative dementias. J. Am. Geriat. Soc. 35: 1127–1129.
4. Volpe BT and Petito CK (1985) Dementia with bilateral medial temporal lobe ischemia. Neurology 35: 1793–1797.
5. Kaplan JG, Katzman R, Horoupian DS et al. (1985) Progressive dementia, visual deficits, amyotrophy, and microinfarcts. Neurology 35: 789–796.

6. Larson EB, Reifler BV, Sumi SM et al. (1986) Diagnostic tests in the evaluation of dementia. Arch. Intern. Med. 146: 1917–1922.
7. Binswanger O (1894) Die Abgrenzung der allgemeinen progressiven Paralyse. Berl. Klin. Wschr. 31: 1103–1105; 1137–1139; 1180–1186.
8. Caplan LR and Schoene WC (1978) Clinical features of subcortical arteriosclerotic encephalopathy (Binswanger's disease). Neurology 28: 1206–1215.
9. Agnoli A, Ruggieri S, Denaro A et al. (1984) White matter disease (Binswanger's encephalopathy) in chronic cerebrovascular disorders. Monogr. Neural. Sci. 11: 144–149.
10. Brun A and Englund E (1986) A white matter disorder in dementia of the Alzheimer type: A pathological study. Ann. Neurol. 19: 253–262.
11. Scheibel AB, Duong T and Tomiyasu U (1987) Denervation microangiopathy in senile dementia, Alzheimer type. Alz. Dis. Assoc. Dis. 1: 19–37.
12. Olszewski J (1965) Subcortical arteriosclerotic encephalopathy. World Neurol. 3: 359–373.
13. Okeda R (1973) Morphometrische Vergleichsuntersuchungen an Hirnarterien bei Binswangerencephalopathie und Hochdruchenencephalopathie. Acta Neuropath. Berl. 26: 23–43.
14. Valentine AR, Moseley IF and Kendall BE (1980) White matter abnormality in cerebral atrophy: Clinicoradiological correlations. J. Neurol. Neurosurg. Psychiat. 43: 139–142.
15. Kingsley DPA and Kendall BE (1978) The value of computed tomography in the evaluation of the enlarged head. Neuroradiology 15: 57–71.
16. Ernest M, Fahn S, Karp J et al. (1974) Normal pressure hydrocephalus and hypertensive cerebrovascular disease. Arch. Neurol. 31: 262–266.
17. Inzitari D, Bracco L, Caparelli R et al. (1984) Cerebrospinal fluid dynamics, white matter degeneration, and mental deterioration in subcortical arteriosclerotic encephalopathy of Binswanger type. Monogr. Neural. Sci. 11: 150–156.
18. Feigin I, Budzilovich G, Weinberg S et al. (1973) Degeneration of white matter in hypoxia, acidosis and edema. J. Neuropathol. Exptl. Neurol. 32: 125–141.
19. Pulsinelli WA and Duffy TE (1979) Local cerebral glucose metabolism during controlled hypoxemia in rats. Science 204: 626–629.
20. Hachinski VC, Potter P and Merskey DM (1987) Leukoaraiosis. Arch. Neurol. 44: 21–23.
21. Crooks LE, Mills CM, Davis PL et al. (1982) Visualisation of cerebral and vascular abnormalities by NMR imaging. Radiology 44: 843–852.
22. Goto K, Ishii N and Fukasawa H (1981) Diffuse white matter disease in the geriatric population. Radiology 141: 687–695.
23. Steingart A, Nachinski VC, Lau C et al. (1987) Cognitive and neurologic findings in subjects with diffuse white matter lucencies on computed tomographic scan (leukoaraiosis). Arch. Neurol. 44: 32–35, 1987.
24. Johnson WK, Davis KR, Buannono FS, Brady TJ, Rosen TJ and Growden JH (1987) Tomography in dementia. Arch. Neurol. 44: 1075–1080.
25. Kertesz A, Black SE, Tokar G et al. (1988) Periventricular and subcortical hyperintensities on magnetic resonance imaging. Arch. Neurol. 45: 404–408.
26. Gupta SR, Naheedy MN, Young JC, Ghobrial M, Rubino FA and Hindo W (1988) Periventricular white matter changes and dementia – clinical, neuropsychological, radiological, and pathological corelation. Arch. Neurol. 45: 637–641.
27. Barclay L (1988) Differential diagnosis of dementing diseases. Age 11: 19–22.
29. Wade JPH, Mirsen TR, Hachinski VC, Fisman M, Lau C and Merskey N (1987) The clinical diagnosis of Alzheimer's disease. Arch. Neurol. 44: 24–29.
28. Hachinski VC, Illiff LD, Zilkha E et al. (1975) Cerebral blood flow in dementia. Arch. Neurol. 32: 632–637.
30. Rosen WG, Terry RD, Fuld PA, Katzman R and Peck A (1980) Pathological verification of ischemic score in differentiation of dementias. Ann. Neurol 7: 486–488.
31. Spitzer RL (ed.) Diagnostic and Statistical Manual of Mental Disorders (1980) 3rd edition, American Psychiatric Association, pp. 127–128.

32. Farber JF, Schmitt FA and Logue PE (1988) Predicting intellectual level from the mini-mental state examination. J. Am. Geriat. Soc. 36: 509–510.
33. Rosen WG, Mohs RC and Davis KL (1984) A new rating scale for Alzheimer's disease. Am. J. Psychiat. 141: 1356–1364.
34. Parnetti L, Ciufetti G, Mercuri M, Lupatelli G and Senin U (1986) The role of haemorrheological factors in the aging brain: Long-term therapy with pentoxifylline ('Trental' 400) in elderly patients with initial mental deterioration. Pharmatherapeutica 4: 617–627.
35. Dominguez D, de Cayaffa CL, Gomensoro J and Aparicio NJ (1977) Modification of psychometric, practical and intellectual parameters in patients with diffuse cerebrovascular insufficiency during prolonged treatment with pentoxifylline: A double-blind, placebo-controlled trial. Pharmatherapeutica 1: 498–506.

The management of chronic cerebral ischaemia

H. Lechner and R. Schmidt
Department of Neurology and Psychiatry, Karl-Franzens University of Graz, Austria

Introduction

Cerebrovascular disease (CVD) has become the third most common cause of death and disability in developed countries. Its clinical symptomatology may present with focal neurological deficits and/or more generalised symptoms such as cognitive impairment, affective and sleep disturbances, vertigo, tinnitus or headache. Therapy during the chronic stage of CVD should be aimed at both prevention of recurrent strokes and improvement of less specific symptoms, which may actually increase the patient's quality of life.

Although the advent of new laboratory and imaging techniques significantly extended the diagnostic potential and pathophysiological insight into cerebral ischaemia, therapy could not keep abreast of this development.

Despite the large number of studies indicating efficacy of medical and non-medical measures, the quality of the predominant part of these trials may be questioned because of non-relevant study design or sample size. This article tries to provide a critical overview on previous literature. In order to evaluate published results a grading system considering the quality of design and the number of patients included in the studies will be used (Table 1). For the assessment of the right sample size Taylor's criteria are applied.

Life-quality improving measures

Medical treatment

A nonuniform group of substances assumed to activate brain metabolism and particularly interfere with neuro-transmission has been indicated to provide benefit in respect to symptoms caused by chronic misery perfusion. Out of the large amount of such 'encephalotrophic' drugs more extensive clinical data are available for ergoloid mesylate, pyrinitol and piracetam.

Ergoloid mesylate is an ergot derivative and consists of a mixture of the methane sulphonates of dihydroergocornine, dihydroergocristine, dihydro-α-ergocryptine and dihydro-ß-ergocryptine, in their natural ratio of 3:3:2:1. In animal studies the

Table 1. Trial grading

Trial type		Grade
Anecdotal report and non randomized trials		I
Randomized	Sample size below Taylor's criteria	II
Randomized double-blind		III
Randomized (double-blind)	Sample size fulfilling Taylor's criteria	IV

substance increased EEG power that had been reduced by hypotension and normalised cortical pO_2 distribution [1]. Thus, a metabolic effect was postulated which would result in an increased capacity of the neuron to maintain a functional steady state, even under conditions when its metabolic tolerance is limited [2]. A number of functional studies support an effect on neuro-transmission. At concentrations of 1–10 nM hydergine in vitro binds to receptors specific for noradrenaline and dopamine [3]. Moreover co-dergocrine mesylate altered the sleep-wakefulness cycle of rats as did 5-hydroxytryptophan [4] and reduced the frequency of high voltage potentials induced by reserpine in cats. A reduction of these waves is indicative of a serotonin agonist effect [5]. In addition a reduction of platelet aggregation has been reported after application of hydergine [6].

The metabolic effects of the substance, its influence on platelets and a reduction of elevated blood pressure have enforced clinical studies on its effect on cerebrovascular disorders. However, most of these trials are uncontrolled and only anecdotal (Table 2). Some of them revealed beneficial effects [7–11]. However, the data of these studies are not conclusive at all, since the authors in most instances provide no control group. Moreover the length of follow-up does not, on the whole, exceed 3 months and the number of patients included is small.

Comparative trials on a more reliable scientific basis [12–15] failed to demonstrate advantages of ergoloid mesylate in comparison to any other treatment. The only exception is the study of Rammohan [16], in which 85% of hydergine treated cases, but only 45% of controls showed remarkable improvement in respect to motor power, speech and mental alertness, after a follow-up of 3 months. However, the study consisted of only 40 stroke patients (20 receiving ergoloid mesylate, 20 generally treated). Besides this small number of cases no comment on the distribution of risk factors in both groups has been provided.

Pyritinol is an encephalotrophic drug which has been indicated to initiate several beneficial metabolic effects. It is thought to improve cerebral glucose utilisation and global as well as regional perfusion values in patients with organic brain-syndromes and brain ischaemia [17–19]. Animal experiments in rats assumed

Table 2. Clinical trials of co-dergocrine in CVD

Study	Substances	Patient type	No.	Follow-up (months)	Effect	Grading
Aradas	Co-dergocrine	Mixed	30	–	+	I
Berselli	Co-dergocrine	Mixed	30	1	+	I
Donnes	Co-dergocrine	Mixed	82	36	+	I
Gross	Co-dergocrine	Stroke	12	–	+	I
Kaiser	Co-dergocrine	Mixed	34	1	+	I
Palleschi	Co-dergocrine	Mixed	25	–	+	I
Mazon	Co-dergocrine	Mixed	50	4	+	I
Rammohan	Co-dergocrine	Stroke	40	3	+	I
Bronzini	Co-dergocrine	Stroke	400	1	–	I
Bochner	Co-dergocrine	Chronic	39	3	–	III
Almici	Co-dergocrine Papaverin	Stroke	192	1	+[a]	II
Otoma	Vinpocetine Ifenprodil Co-dergocrine	Mixed	288	6	–	I
Santambrogio	Co-dergocrine Co-dergocrine + Dexamethasone Co-dergocrine + Mannitol Placebo	Stroke	300	12	–	I

[a] Not indicated, if difference is significant.

interactions with the cholinergic system of the brain, since the application of pyritinol induces an increase in both the presynaptic choline uptake and the postsynaptic cyclic guanosine monophosphate, which is known to act as a second messenger in the cholinergic system [20,21]. In respect to cerebrovascular disorders an improvement of red cell aggregability and flexibility under pyrotoxin treatment attracts attention [22].

Although a number of clinical trials exist proving the efficacy of the drug in organic brain syndromes of different origins, little is known about the effect of pyritinol in patients suffering from cerebral ischaemia. A study [23] summarised the results of a series of randomised double-blind trials consisting of 458 patients presenting with different types of cerebrovascular disease. Significant differences between verum- and placebo-treated groups have been reported for global improvement rating (67% vs. 53%) and subjective symptoms (59% vs. 47%) following a therapy of 8 weeks. EEG improvements almost paralleled clinical amelioration. However, as can be seen from the numbers in parentheses, the differences were rather small and there may be criticism with respect to both the items considered and the inhomogeneity of disorders of included patients. Positive results in favour of pyrinitol were also described by other authors with regard to

Table 3. Clinical trials for pyrinitol in CVD

Study	Patient type	No.	Significant effect	Follow-up (months)	Grading
Dolce (1988)	Post-stroke	50	SCAG NUDS Digit-span CGI	3	III
Arjundas (1987)	Stroke	71	Memory	2	III
Tazaki (1980)	Mixed	458	Global improvement (67 vs. 53%) Subjective symptom improvement (59 vs. 47%)	2	III

cognitive [24,25] and effective disturbances [24] investigating small samples of patients in a randomised fashion (Table 3).

Piracetam, a derivative of aminobutyric acid is also proposed to provide a beneficial effect in the post-stroke period. However, this assumption is based on improvements of cerebral blood flow and regional glucose metabolism [26] under treatment (Table 4) rather than on clinical data [19,27,28]. Another substance, which promises to be efficacious in patients with mental impairment based on both cerebral ischaemia and primary degenerative disease is phosphatidylserin. This agent is an acidic phospholipid present in biological membranes and is thought to induce cerebral glucose accumulation as well as an elevation of the striatal and cortical acetyl-choline content. Clinical effects have been claimed in both open [29] and controlled trials [30,31]. However, the effects were only modest and the number of patients was again small.

Table 4. Effccts of piracetam on functional parameters

Study	Patient type	Parameter
Heiss (1983)	Acute stroke	LCMRGI $P < 0.05$ in infarct areas (10–27%)
Depresseux (1986)	Acute stroke	CBF $CMRO_2$ $P < 0.05$–0.008 in infarct areas (7.5–13.2%)
OTT (1988)	MID	CBF $P < 0.001$ (13%)
Sitzer (1981)	Acute stroke	EEG changes improved

Pentoxifylline (PTX), a haemorheologically active substance has been frequently reported to increase global and regional cerebral blood flow [32]. Consistent with functional improvement several studies indicate beneficial effects of PTX on a variety of clinical symptoms and psychometric test results mainly when administered for a longer time. Eight of these trials [33–40] were performed in a double-blind randomised fashion.

Calcium channel blockers have been hypothesised to counteract the mechanism of neuronal cell death based on chronic cerebral minor perfusion in two ways. They are assumed to reduce elevated ischaemia related intracellular calcium content in brain tissue and smooth muscle cells resulting from impeded ATP-sodium-potassium transport causing a lowering of the membrane potential. This in turn opens the calcium channels and leads to an influx of calcium ions. Inhibition of this process reduces the activation of autocatalytic mechanisms based on the development of free arachidonic acid and radicals respectively reduces post-ischemic hypoperfusion by relaxation of the vascular smooth muscles. A large number of animal studies have been performed indicating efficacy of nimodipine after experimental brain ischaemia. Positive effects were objectivated with respect to post-ischemic cerebral blood flow [41–46], ischemic volume [46,47], neurologic outcome and mortality [47,48] as well as EEG-improvement [45,49,50]. Encouraged by experimental data several trials using nimodipine in chronic CVD at dosages between 30 and 120 mg per day have been initiated. Except for one recent study [51] nimodipine provided significant improvement of neuropsychological test results in comparison to placebo in all of these studies (Table 5). However, none of these studies can be unequivocally accepted, since the treated groups in part consist of etiologically nonuniform groups [52,53] and in part, the sample size is to small to allow conclusive results.

Non-medical treatment

Non-medical measures aimed at improving quality of life are occupied with both recovery of persistent neuropsychological deficits following cerebral ischaemia, and social reintegration. Rehabilitation efforts are provided by a number of specialists such as physical and speech therapists, social workers and physicians. However, the question arises, whether such rehabilitation programmes significantly improve the patient's outcome over those of the natural history of recovery. This question cannot be conclusively answered at present since only a small number of studies have been published comparing rehabilitation programme groups of patients with those routinely cared for in a prospective randomised manner. Most of these trials [54–57] report statistical benefit for activities of daily living and motility but no influence on mortality or medical complications. However, controversial results have been reported by others [58–60]. One of the main flaws in the mentioned trials is that the type and intensity of therapeutic measures are poorly documented. Moreover, almost no information exists about particular strategies to inpatient rehabilitation [61]. Language and cognitive therapies include a variety of approaches, but their values have not yet been clarified in an appropriate manner. A recent review [62] on the literature of rehabilitation programmes proposed a

Table 5. Clinical trials on the efficacy of nimodipine in chronic CVD

Study	Patient type	No.	Follow-up (months)	Dose (mg/day)	Significant effects	Grading
Zamperini (1984)	CVI	23	2	30	SCAG Token Copy of drawing visual de-nomination	I
Cosmi (1986)	CVI	32	3	30	SCAG Vertigo Well-being	I
Maio (1987)	VI	32	3	30	Digit-span Corsi block Tapping test Total score	I
Dycka (1986)	Mixed VD + SDAT	1000	3	30/60	SCAG Trailmarking	III
Menazzi (1984)	CVI	86	3	30	Wechseler Subtests	III
Dorn (1985)	CVI	68	3	–	SCAG Bf-S-score Labyrinth-test Trail-masking	III
Held (1985)	CVI	24	3	90	Digit-span Symbol digit Span	III
Agnoli (1986)	CVI	12	1	120	CBF attention short term memory	
Besson (1988)	MID	20	6	30	Neg.	III
Tobares (1988)	VD	33	6	90	SPMSQ Digit-span SCAG	III
Fischhof (1988)	Mixed	130	3	–	SCAG SKT	III

randomised study, in which one half of the patients, matched for age, sex, side of stroke and severity of neurological and functional impairment, would receive rehabilitation and the other half would not. Interesting end points would be: the final level of functional outcome, the time required to reach the outcome goal and the number of patients discharged home versus institutional care. Another important requirement will be the use of refined specific measures of function as has been indicated by Dobkin [61]. The impact of treatment of depression, frequently occurring during the post-stroke period [63] on the rehabilitation process has also not been investigated yet, although it may provide a valuable support on the way to the rehabilitation goal.

Cerebrovascular risk factors

The control of risk factors for stroke is most likely of crucial importance for both improvement of life quality and secondary prevention. As has been indicated by the Framingham study and other investigations, arterial hypertension, cardiac disease and diabetes mellitus are the major predicting factors for ischemic stroke [64,65]. The association of other factors like elevated serum cholesterol or cigarette smoking, obesity, alcohol consumption or physical activity is far less clear or consistent [66]. These parameters may play a supportive role in the pathogenesis of primary risk factors rather than per se increase cerebrovascular risk. Increased risk has also been observed with the presence of high haematocrit and serum fibrinogen levels [67–69]. The latter factor seems to interact with atherogenesis and thrombus formation. Reliable data on the effect of risk factor control in primary stroke prevention exist for arterial hypertension only. The United States Hypertension Detection and Follow-up Program involving nearly 11,000 persons with high blood pressure reported a significantly lower mortality than in those given standard care (Hypertension Detection and Follow-up Program Cooperative Research Group [70]). Two large multi-center trials confirm the reduction of stroke risk by approximately 50% in mild to moderate hypertensive subjects under treatment [71]. There has been a tendency to assume that the decline in stroke mortality in the United States and in western European countries can be attributed to an increase in the proportion of patients receiving antihypertensive treatment [72]. However, a recent publication [73] performed an analysis of 9 randomised trials and suggested a 6–16% stroke reduction. Although clinical studies may underestimate the benefit of treatment even epidemiological data indicate that only between 16 and 25% of the overall mortality decline can be explained by the benefit of antihypertensive drugs. Despite the lack of prospective data on the extent of treatment efficacy for other risk factors, one will probably have to consider the control of risk factors for stroke as an effective measure for primary prevention. Although it would be logical for the same to be true for the prevention of recurrent strokes there has as yet been no clinical trial performed that would really support the latter consideration.

Secondary prevention

Medical treatment

Previously the efficacy of three types of substances i.e., antiplatelet agents, haemorheologically active substances and anticoagulants, has been examined in prospective randomised studies.

Antiplatelet therapy

The efficacy of platelet anti-aggregating substances has been studied extensively but the number of trials performed in a double-blind randomised fashion is small. Drugs submitted to such studies were aspirin, sulfinpyrazone, dipyridamole and recently ticlopidine. Most extensive attention was attracted to acetylsalicylic acid (ASA) and although there still remains some controversy in respect to the real efficacy, sex differences and the proper dose, it became the standard preventive therapy in patients with a high risk of recurrent strokes.

The inhibition of the aggregation-release reaction of platelets has been related to a blocking of the transformation of hydrolysed arachidonic acid to labile cyclic endoperoxide forms of prostaglandins PGG_2 and PGH_7 [74].

Placebo-controlled trials. The first larger double-blind study on the preventive potential of aspirin was started in 1972 by Fields and indicated a decreased risk of cerebral and retinal infarction by 30% and a combined infarct-death rate of 28% after 2 years. However, there was no significant difference between the ASA and the placebo group probably due to the small number of patients included. Significance in favour of aspirin treatment was mainly revealed in patients with a history of multiple TIAs.

One year after the publication of Fields' study, the Canadian Cooperative Study Group [75] also reported a beneficial effect of aspirin on stroke prevention, although this was only true for men. The investigators compared ASA, sulfinpyrazone, the combination of these agents and placebo. They indicated a 48% stroke and death reduction for men (62% for those with no history of myocardial infarction). Sulfinpyrazone was not efficacious.

Three Scandinavian studies; the Danish Cooperative [76], the Swedish [77] and the Danish very low dose after carotid endarterectomy trial [78], failed to demonstrate a beneficial effect of aspirin. In the first Danish trial 13% in each group died or had recurrent strokes. However, there was a risk reduction of almost 10% for myocardial infarcts. In Boysen's low dose trial [78] aspirin reduced the overall risk by 11%. In both studies the lack of statistical significance may be a question of small sample size rather than a principle one. The main difference of the Swedish trial in comparison to most other studies was the inclusion of patients with only minor or major strokes. Gent [79] in an accompanying editorial emphasises the selection of this special group and derives that the effect of ASA may be different in patients with reversible ischemic deficits than in those with completed strokes.

Bousser [80], however, in the 'AICLA' trial in part also studied completed stroke patients, but unfortunately provided no separate data analysis for this cohort. The largest placebo-controlled study evaluating the efficacy of ASA in two different dosages (300 mg and 1200 mg/day) was the UK-TIA study [81] including 2435 individuals. The odds of patients suffering from one or more of four possible endpoints (nonfatal myocardial infarction, nonfatal major stroke, vascular death, or nonvascular death) were 18% less in the two serum groups in comparison to placebo.

A few studies determined the prophylactic potential of ASA combined with other substances.

ASA plus dipyridamole was the subject of two large multi-centre trials, the American-Canadian Cooperative Trial [82] and the European Stroke Prevention Study [83] (ESPS) including 890 resp. 2500 patients randomly selected. In the American study the results of life table analysis of aspirin-only and aspirin plus persantine groups were identical. The ESPS reports a 33% benefit of the ASA-persantine group in comparison to placebo, which is not higher than the benefit indicated by other studies for ASA alone. Thus, it is unlikely that dipyridamole adds protection as it has also been emphasised by Bousser and a Spanish group [84].

Comparative, not placebo-controlled trials. Three studies compared the efficacy of sulfinpyrazone and dipyridamole with that of ASA. The trial with the largest sample was the American-Canadian Cooperative Study including 890 individuals. The endpoint results did not demonstrate any difference between ASA alone and ASA plus dipyridamole treated groups. A Spanish trial [84] and Bousser's results accordingly emphasised that dipyridamole does not add protection to ASA treatment in respect to stroke recurrence. Candelise [85] in his studies evaluated the relative efficacy of sulfinpyrazone and ASA. He confirmed the benefit of ASA for men (53% risk reduction for further events) and demonstrated a favourable but not significant trend of sulfinpyrazone in females. However, the number of patients included was only 124 and the clinical selection criteria were not uniform enough for such a small cohort.

Metaanalysis of data. Concern has been expressed with respect to the relatively small sample size in all previous studies on antiplatelet agents. Therefore, two metaanalyses of randomised trials integrating data of multiple studies were performed in order to increase the statistical power. The first report [86] analysed seven studies and indicated a nonsignificant 15% reduction of recurrent strokes regarding ASA alone, but a 39% decline of recidivation when combined treatment (ASA plus sulfinpyrazone or dipyridamole; $P < 0.05$) was administered. The second and more complete analysis (Antiplatelet trialist collaboration [87]) summarised 25 trials including 29,000 patients. In order to provide comparability of data the authors calculated the observed minus expected number of failures in the actively treated groups. The calculation tends to give a negative result if treatment

Table 6. Structure, grading and observed (O) – expected (E) number of vascular events (stroke, MI, death) in randomized trials on antiplatelet treatment (modified Antiplatelet Trialist Collaboration)

Study	Patient type	No.	Agent(s)	Dosage (mg/day)	Follow-up (yrs)	Trial grading	O–E events	P
I. Placebo-controlled, single substance								
Danish very low dose TEA	TEA	301	ASA	50–100	2	III	2.5	N.S.
Swedish COS	CS	305	ASA	1500	2	III	2.4	N.S.
Acheson	TIA, CS	169	DP	400–800	2	III	2.4	N.S.
German TIA	TIA, AF	60	ASA	1500	2	III	–0.5	N.S.
Toronto	CS	290	SP	1000	3	III	–1.5	N.S.
Tennesse	TIA, MS	148	SP	800	6	III	–1.7	N.S.
Danish COS	TIA, AF	203	ASA	1000	2	III	–2.4	N.S.
MAC Master	CS	447	SP	600	2	III	–3.6	N.S.
Fields (AITIA)	TIA, AF	303	ASA	1300	1	III	–4.8	N.S.
UK-TIA	TIA, AF	2435	ASA	1200, 300	2	IV	–19.5	0.02
ESPS	TIA, CS	2500	ASA+DP	975+225	2	IV	–41.0	0.000
II. Placebo-controlled comparative								
Canadian COS	TIA, AF, MS	585	DP ASA ASA+SP	800 1300 1300+800	2	III	1.1	N.S.
Toulouse	TIA, MS	440	ASA ASA+DP	900 900+150	3	III	–2.5	N.S.
Bousser	TIA, CS	604	ASA ASA+DP	990 990+225	3	III	–11.2	0.01
All trials (active proportion: 4081)							–80.2	0.000

Abbreviations: COS = Cooperative study, TEA = Thromboendarterectomy, CS = Completed stroke, AF = Amaurosis fugax, MS = Mild stroke, ASA = Acetylsalicylic acid, DP = Dipyridamole, SP = Sulfinpyrazone.

works, and an equally balanced trial is equal in size to about half the patients protected. An updated version modified for the grading of each trial is provided in Table 6. Out of 14 studies, analysis revealed beneficial effects of ASA in 10. Statistical significance has been reached in only 3 of them. However, it is of importance that these studies included the highest number of patients and were sufficiently designed (score IV on our grading scale). The latter is supportive to the preventive efficacy of ASA in CVD. The overall data analysis as performed by the Antiplatelet Trialists Collaboration yielded a 30% reduction of vascular mortality and fatal vascular events under treatment with antiplatelet substances. The beneficial effect was more pronounced for myocardial infarction than for cerebrovascular disease. This finding merits attention, because cardiac disease accounts for a large proportion of deaths in such a population [88]. Anti-aggregating therapy is able to reduce the recurrence of nonfatal and fatal vascular events by about a quarter among patients with evidence of cerebrovascular disease, but there still remain some open questions with respect to the use of aspirin in secondary prevention. One is the optimal dose, another the possible unresponsiveness of females.

Dose dependency of ASA. The optimal dose of ASA is still undetermined. It has been demonstrated that 40 mg aspirin may inhibit hyper-aggregability of thrombocytes sufficiently in patients with cerebrovascular disease. However, the individual variability of this effect was relatively large and the only trial that tested such a low dose failed to demonstrate a significant effect [78]. The United Kingdom TIA aspirin trial [81] for the first time evaluated the effect of both low (300 mg daily) and high (1200 mg daily) dose ASA in a prospective manner. The authors conclude that the overall reduction of vascular events during follow-up was 18% but data analysis revealed no significant difference between the two dose groups although patients receiving low-dose aspirin had less gastroenteric side effects.

Efficacy of ASA and gender. The Canadian Cooperative study [89] for the first time indicated that ASA might be effective in men only. This may be due to a better prognosis for females with threatened stroke, but could have been also a type I statistical error caused by the low ratio of women included [90]. Although the latter is possible, the results of a recent study [91] showing an influence of testosterone on the inhibitory effect of aspirin on the aggregability of blood platelets has to be considered an important finding which may provide an explanation of the relative lack of aspirin response in women. This would implicate the use of different antiplatelet drugs or a combination of agents in females.

Ticlopidine. Ticlopidine is a relatively new anti-aggregating substance and was the subject of two large multi-centred trials (The Canadian-American ticlopidine study – CATS [92], and The Ticlopidine Aspirin Stroke Study – TASS [93]). The TASS revealed a higher risk reduction for ticlopidine than for ASA. Toxicity, however, emerged as an important concern. Reversible leukopenia occurred in approximately 1% of ticlopidine treated patients. Intracerebral haemorrhage during therapy was found in only 2 ticlopidine individuals and often similar in controls.

Haemorheologically effective substances

Pentoxifylline reduces blood viscosity by increasing cell flexibility and decreasing the fibrinogen concentration of blood which per se may increase the aggregability of erythrocytes [94]. The agent was first introduced for therapy of intermittent claudication and is also thought to be efficacious in different types of cerebrovascular disease. Herskovitz in 1981 [95] provided a comparison of the outcome of two TIA groups matched for age, sex and hypertension receiving either pentoxifylline or ASA plus dipyridamole and reported a significant effect of the drug to prevent recurrent TIAs. The incidence of completed strokes was similar in both groups but lower than in historical controls. In a second attempt with larger samples he confirmed previous results [96]. The beneficial effect of pentoxifylline has also been supported by another trial [97] comparing TIA patients with good therapeutical compliance and a non-compliant control group. The recurrence rate of pentoxifylline treated patients was 8.6% but 38% in controls. This difference reached statistical significance. However, it has to be considered that patients with bad compliance may also have neglected the importance of risk factors for stroke during follow-up. It may therefore be argued, that although both groups were comparable for risk factors at the entry into the study they might have been different during follow-up.

Anticoagulant therapy

Anticoagulants are predominantly used for secondary stroke prevention in patients with atrial fibrillation which occurs in approximately 20% of hospitalised stroke patients. It is hypothesised that anticoagulants interfere with the process of thromboembolism and reduce the risk of embolisation particularly to the brain. Although it has been embedded in clinical practice that the latter is possible, it has again not been proven by randomised trials. There have been numerous comparative studies based on reviews of case books indicating beneficial effects of immediate anticoagulation after cerebral ischaemia. However, most of them ignored coexistent risk factors which might have also influenced the outcome of patients and/or controls [98]. Recently a cooperative study compared stroke patients with non-rheumatic atrial fibrillation of 2 centres with different treatment policies over 5 years. Anticoagulated patients did not fare better than those not receiving anticoagulants [99]. These results are in good shape with 2 other studies also reporting negative results [100,101]. A major problem with these drugs is their potential to cause haemorrhagic infarcts or even intracerebral haemorrhage. However, the risk of anticoagulating therapy, estimated at 4.3 haemorrhagic complications per 100 treatment years [102] is very similar to the risk of first stroke in patients with atrial fibrillation (4.5 per 100 treatment years) as indicated by the Framingham study [103]. Controversy of results emphasises the necessity of a large randomised long-term trial in order to evaluate the efficacy of anticoagulating therapy in patients with possible cardiac sources for cerebral infarcts.

Surgical treatment

Atherosclerotic occlusive disease of the major brain-supplying arteries can be observed in more than 50% of stroke patients [104]. The literature indicates annual stroke indices (number of events/duration of risk exposure) from 0 to 12.5 for carotid stenosis [105–107] and a 5–10% risk of recurrent strokes per year with the presence of haemodynamically significant occlusions [108].

The first surgical therapeutic approaches were initiated in the early fifties [109] and over the following decades carotid endarterectomy and EC/IC arterial bypass were among the most common vascular procedures performed [110,111]. However, although widely applied, there remained some concern among neurologists and neurosurgeons that both techniques might not necessarily benefit the operated patient.

The emerging criticism during the last 10 years was the reason for performing the International EC/IC Bypass Study [112] involving 71 centers all over the world and the value of carotid endarterectomy was called to question.

The EC/IC bypass study

The trial included 1377 patients randomly assigned to surgical or medical treatment, followed them for an average of 55.8 months and was performed to test whether an EC/IC bypass would decrease the frequency of recurrent transient ischemic attacks or other types of cerebrovascular disease. The results showed no effect of surgery compared to acetylsalicylic acid treatment alone in preventing cerebral ischemic events. Even separate analysis of data with respect to subgroups of patients that have been considered to particularly benefit from the procedure such as those with internal carotid or middle cerebral artery occlusion and continuing transient ischemic attacks [113] failed to demonstrate any effectiveness of the bypass in comparison to medical treatment. The study also provides data on the clinical improvement of patients developing serious ipsilateral cerebral infarction. Based on the observation that cerebral blood flow and metabolism in the region of cerebral infarction may increase after bypass surgery some groups postulated a better clinical outcome after recurrent strokes for patients with an EC/IC bypass than for those without [114–116]. However, this hypothesis could not be supported by the study, since the comparison of the final functional status of medically and surgically treated individuals after the first major ipsilateral ischemic stroke revealed no statistically significant difference. As has been stated by Cote and Caron [117] one of the remaining, but still unproven, indications for a bypass application may be the evidence of internal carotid occlusion and misery perfusions detected by PET not responding to medical therapy. Although the study may have been the best randomly controlled trial of a surgical procedure yet performed, some criticisms have been made by surgeons, who actively performed EC/IC bypass operations outside the study [118,119]. The most striking reply was that data may be distorted by not taking into account the large group of 2572 patients that have been operated on during the observation period of the trial without being included. However, reanalysis of the study data failed to demonstrate that not considering these patients influenced the results [120].

Carotid endarterectomy

Carotid endarterectomy is a very logical surgical procedure and is directed towards removal of ulcerative atherosclerotic plaques and haemodynamically effective vessel occlusion. Reviewing the data of the National Hospital Discharge Survey, the Veterans Administration Hospitals and the Departments of Army, Air Force and Navy in the United States, Dyken and Pokras [121] indicated an exponential increase in the number of endarterectomies per year performed between 1972 and 1982. The number of operations in Europe are much lower, but were continuously increasing from year to year [122]. However, it is difficult to understand why a procedure that may cause relatively high numbers of peri-operative stroke and

Table 7. Stroke and death following TEA: Comparison of study and expected frequency (in accordance to Warlow)

Study	Trial grading	No. patients	Follow-up (months)	Stroke and/ or death	Expected stroke and/or death	
					10%/Annum	7.4%/Annum
Siekert	I	32	24	12	6.4	4.7
Heyman	I	49	40	21	16.3	12.1
Young	I	104	36	19	31.2	23.1[a]
Thompson	I	293	42	91	102.6	75.9[b]
Nunn	I	170	39	58	55.2	40.9
Mungas	I	80	13	11	8.7	6.4
Stanford	I	128	20	11	21.3	15.8[a]
Park	I	65	32	22	17.3	12.8
Owens	I	113	28	8	26.4	19.5[a]
Erikson	I	32	21	7	5.6	4.1
Parkin	I	20	48	5	8.0	5.9[a]
Muronnen	I	82	20	18	13.9	10.3
Fields	II	169	42	45	59.2	43.8[b]
Shaw	II	20	156	15	26	19.2[a]

[a]Study with better outcome than the expected 7.4% and 10% stroke and death rate; [b]Study with better outcome than the expected 7.4% stroke and death rate.

death (24.4–25%) has been forced so much during the last 2 decades, especially since there have been no reliable data revealing that it is really advantageous to medical therapy. Besides numerous, mostly retrospective and non-randomised trials so far only 2 prospective random studies have been published [123,124] and only one of them was a multi-center trial [123]. The benefit of endarterectomy reported by several non-randomised studies has been based on the comparison of their surgical groups with historical controls or with controls not randomly selected. Besides these doubts on the data Warlow additionally disarmed the accuracy of these results when comparing the 'expected number of annual strokes and deaths' with the annual risk without surgery indicated as 10% in the Canadian Co-operative ASA Study or as 7.4% in the American Joint Study. In 50% of the studies evaluated, patients who underwent surgery fared worse than expected (Table 7). The explanation Warlow gave with respect to the possible misinterpretation of the data was that the authors often excluded minor strokes during follow-up in the surgical group, selected the worst natural history studies for comparison and refrained from adding the complication rate of angiography to the entire risk of surgery. In another attempt to evaluate the efficacy of the procedure in patients with ipsilateral TIA, PRIND or minor strokes in the carotid territory, Jonas [125] analysed the data provided by previous literature for intact months of patient survival (IMPS). The IMPS ratio is the ratio between the total number of months during which patients of a cohort had not been suffering from strokes or deaths and the maximum amount of months this population could have been without complications. On the basis of this index the required annual stroke and death rate for surgery to 'break even' with nonsurgical care has been calculated for those non-random studies that provide data on follow-up and operative stroke morbidity and mortality [126–128]. There was only one study population [126] whose outcome might have been better than the one indicated by the 2 randomised trials providing data for controls (American Joint Study [124]).

As indicated above only two prospective randomised trials have been published to date. The first one was performed already in the 1960s and consisted of 316 patients with transient ischemic attacks randomly allocated to surgical or nonsurgical treatment and followed them between 7 and 63 months (42 months mean). Both groups were comparable for sex, age and vascular risk. In the surgical group 11.2% of patients died or had nonfatal stroke during the peri-operative period. During the follow-up 3 patients suffered from fatal, 3 from non-fatal strokes and 20 died of other causes. In the nonsurgical group 10 out of 147 patients had nonfatal, 10 fatal strokes and 18 subjects died from other causes. The overall stroke death rate of the endarterectomy population was therefore 27% vs. 26% in the control cohort. Recurrent TIAs were reported as 38% and 54.5% in the surgical and nonsurgical group. This difference was not of statistical significance, however. The only significance in favour of surgery was found in the percentage of asymptomatic survivors. Although one may derive some advantages of surgery in comparison to medical treatment by these data, we agree with the suggestions of Warlow that the study is far from being conclusive. The major reasons are the small sample of patients in each group, the short follow-up, the inclusion of TIA in the vertebrobasilar territory, the lack of a life-table analysis and the improvement of present medical therapeutic possibilities (control of hypertension, anti-aggregating substances) that may today cause a better outcome for the nonsurgical group. The second prospective randomised trial available was performed by Shaw from 1965–1978 and was published in 1984. This study includes only 20 surgically and 21 nonsurgically treated patients with either TIA or minor stroke. There were only 6 strokes and 30% death during the follow-up of 77 months in the surgical group, but 15 strokes and 75% death in the nonsurgical group, that had been followed for a mean of 72.2 months. However, the peri-operative stroke and death rate was 35% and based on the IMPS analysis, operated patients had thus a less favourable outcome than controls. The question arises as to whether surgery may be of benefit, if the patients are followed for a longer period of time. Although the latter is possible, one should consider the relatively high frequency, ranging from 10–22% [129–131] of restenosis after endarterectomy, that again may increase the risk of operated patients being the victim of recurrent strokes. Therefore a more parallel course of stroke and death curves of surgical vs. nonsurgical groups after some years appears to be more likely than a crossing one. All of these controversies in respect to endarterectomy make the performance of the procedure uncertain and lead to an increasing demand for a prospective randomised multi-center trial satisfying the sample size requirements that have been indicated by Taylor [132] as sufficient for stroke prevention studies. Two such trials are on the way: the European Carotid Surgery Trial since 1982 and the North American Symptomatic Carotid Endarterectomy Trial since 1987 [133].

Conclusion

Therapy of chronic cerebrovascular disease is based on encephalotrophic substances, which are assumed to improve unspecific symptomatology and cognitive deterioration, and medical and surgical measures for secondary prevention. Out of 98 clinical studies reviewed in this article only 6 reached score IV in our grading system indicating highest quality of study design and inclusion of statistically sufficient numbers of patients. Four of these trials studied antiplatelet substances (ESPS, UK-TIA aspirin trial, CATS and TASS). The 2 other studies are the Hypertension Detection and Follow-up Program and the EC/IC Bypass Trial.

No comparable study has been performed for any of encephalotrophic substances. Although beneficial effects are repeatedly reported for ergoloid mesylate, pyrinitol, piracetam, nimodipine and PTX the reliability of data may be questioned for several reasons: 1. It is unclear if functional changes such as improvement of EEG changes, oxygen and/or glucose metabolism or cerebral blood flow, which are suggested to verify the efficacy of most of these drugs are really accompanied by clinical benefit; 2. the biological mechanism(s) on which the effectiveness of these substances is based is (are) not fully understood; 3. their therapeutic efficacy on relevant clinical symptomatology is, if actually present, only modest; and 4. the sample size was too small in all available studies.

Reduction and control of cerebrovascular risk factors is most likely effective for both treatment goals in chronic CVD. However, its efficacy has only been established for arterial hypertension.

Antiplatelet substances are the therapy of choice for secondary prevention. The benefit of ASA is well established. Low-dose administration should be performed, since the UK-TIA ASA study indicated comparable reduction of vascular events for the groups receiving either low or high dose aspirin, but less side effects in the former group. Ticlopidine is assumed to provide an even higher preventive effect on the patient irrespective of gender. However, more severe side effects in comparison to ASA can be expected. The use of PTX is a promising approach in prevention of recurrent cerebral ischaemia. However, a large enough multi-center trial has not yet been performed. Long-term anticoagulation although embeeded in clinical practice, was the subject of only a few studies, mostly including miscellaneous groups of cardiac patients and small sample size. The same is true for thromboendarterectomy, the use of which is based on predominantly anecdotal reports, but only 2 randomised trials with several methodological flaws. The value of the procedure will hopefully be evaluated by two large ongoing multi-centre trials.

Patient selection in previous therapeutic studies was based on clinical data alone. Additional information with respect to the aetiology and type of cerebral infarction probably provided by new imaging techniques such as MRI, SPECT and/or PET could help to better specify treatment groups. Future research considering such information could lead to a more pathogenetic-related therapy of stroke patients and will hopefully induce more specific regimens for better defined samples of stroke patients.

References

1. Wiernsperger N, Gygox P and Danzeisen M (1978) Cortical PO_2 distribution during oligemic hypotension and its pharmacological modification. Arzneim. Forsch. (Drug Res.) 28: 768–770.
2. Meier-Ruge W, Enz A, Gygax P, Henzinker O, Iwangoff P and Reichlmeier K (1975) Experimental pathology in basic research of the ageing brain. In: Gershon and Raskin (eds.) Ageing. Vol. 2, pp. 55–126.
3. Goldstein M, Lew J, Hata F and Liebermann A (1978) Binding interactions of ergot alkaloids with monoaminergic receptors in the brain. Gerontology 24(1): 76–85.
4. Loew DM and Spiegel R (1976) Polygraphic sleep studies in rats and humans. Their use in psychopharmacological research. Arzneim. Forsch. (Drug Res) 26: 1032–1035.
5. Jouvet M (1972) The role of monoamines and acetylcholine containing neurons in the regulation of the sleep-waking cycle. Ergeb. Physiol. 64: 166–307.
6. Perez, Sanchez M, Rocha, Lasas E, Pico M, Cabezuelo A and Fernandez MT (1978) In: Garsi E (ed.) Xth Congresso Nae Gerontol. Geriatr. Madrid, pp. 490–494.
7. Gross D, Leuterer W and Matthiesen G (1952) Aktive Apoplexiebehandlung. Munch. Med. Wschr. 35: 1734–1738.
8. Palleschi M (1976) Cerebrovascular sufficiency in its multiple aspects, observations using derivates of ergot. Clinica (Bologna) 32: 29–35.
9. Kaiser G and Tschabitscher H (1956) Erfahrungen mit Hydergin in der Behandlung zerebraler Durchblutungsstorungen im höheren Alter. Wr. Klin. Wschr. 9: 150–154.
10. Berselli L and Ferracini (1965) The treatment of cerebrovascular accidents. Clinica Bologna 25: 66–75.
11. Aradas A (1965) Treatment of cerebral circulation disorders with dihydrogenated alkaloids of ergot of rye administered intravenously in repeated doses. G. Geront. 11: 677–682.
12. Bochner F, Eadic MJ and Tyrer JH (1973) Use of ergot preparation (Hydergine) in the convalescent phase of stroke. J. Amer. Geriat. Soc. 21: 10–17.
13. Bronzini A, Michetti A and Barkieri R (1967) Therapie der akuten Hirngefäßerkrankungen mit der Kombination Dihydroergocornin, Dihydroergocristin und Dihydroergokryptin plus Novocain. Clin. ter. 41: 515–522.
14. Santambrogio S, Martinotti R, Sardella F, Porro F and Randazzo A (1978) Is there a real treatment for stroke? Clinical and statistical comparison of different treatments in 300 patients. Stroke 9: 130–132.
15. Viala JJ, Bourrat C and Site N (1974) Le prognostic a court terme des accidents vascculaires cerebraux. Lyon Med. 231: 815–819.
16. Rammohan G, Veni AK, Reddy KK, Jamaluddin and Bhatnagar RC (1985) Management of acute ischemic cerebrovascular episodes with parenteral and oral dihydro-ergotoxine mesylate with follow-up for 3 months. Med. Surg. 25: 20A–20B.
17. Becker K and Hoyer S (1966) Hirnstoffwechseluntersuchungen unter der Behandlung von Pyrithioxin. Deutsche Zeitschrift für Nervenheilkunde, 188: 200–209.
18. Hoyer S, Oesterreich K and Stoll KD (1977) Effects of Pyritinol-HCl on blood flow and oxidative metabolism of the brain in patients with dementia. Arzneitmittel-Forschung (Drug Res.) 27: 671–674.
19. Herrschaft H (1978) Die Wirkung von Pyritinol auf die Gehirndurchblutung des Menschen. Munch. Med. Wschr. 39: 1263–1268.
20. Martin K and Vyas S (1987) Increase in acetylcholine concentration in the brain of 'old' rats following treatment with pyrithoxin (Encephabol) Br. J. Pharm. 90: 561–565.
21. Pavlik A, Benesova O and Dlohozkova N (1987) Effects of nootropic drugs on brain cholinergic and dopaminergic transmission. Activas Nervosa Superior Praha 29: 62–65.
22. Kiesewetter H, Jung F and Schneider R (1984) Rheologische Wirkung von Pyrinitol nach einmaliger intravenöser Infusion von 400 mg bei rheologisch auffälligen Probanden. Internen Bericht, Merck.
23. Tazaki G, Omae T, Kuomaru S, Ontono E, Hasagania K, Nori A, Kurihara N, Kutsusawa N and Okada T (1980) Clinical effect of encephabol (pyritinol) in the treatment of cerebrovascular disorders. I. Int. Med. Res. pp. 118–126.

24. Dolce G, Zylberman MR, Fontana M and Paroni-Sterbini GL (1989) The effect of an encephalotrophic drug on the rehabilitation phase of post-stroke hemiplegia. In: Maurer K and Wurtman R (eds.) Organic brain disorders. 1st European Congress of Neurology, Prague 1988. Vieweg Verlag, Braunschweig, pp. 37–46.
25. Arjundas G, Sultana SM and Natarajan V (1987) Influence of an encephalotrophic drug on higher nervous function of stroke patients. In: Higher Nervous Functions. Int. Symposium during the 7th Asian Oceanian Congress of Neurology, Bali. Vieweg Verlag Braunschweig, pp. 121–130.
26. Depresseux JC, Salmon E, Sadzot N, Cornette M and Franck G: Evaluation of the effect of piracetam on CBF and $CMRO_2$ in acute stroke patients using PET and 15 Oxygen. Int. Congress on Senile Dementias 86, Paris.
27. Sitzer G and Matz D (1981) Die Wertigkeit hirnelektrischer Untersuchungen in der Rehabilitation des ischämischen zerebralen Insultes, insbesondere unter Berücksichtigung der toposelektiven Ableitung. Int. Kongress über hematologische und metabolische Aspekte von Piracetam. Heidelberg, pp. 171–179.
28. Herrmann WM and Kern U (1987) Nootropika: Wirkungen und Wirksamkeit. Nervenarzt 58: 358–364.
29. Castellani A, Colafelice M and Perbellini D (1978) Clinical experiments with brain cortex phospholipids in psychogeriatrics. Acta Neurol. 33(3): 217–229.
30. Savoldi F, Nappi G, Martignoni E and Bono G (1978) Brain phospholipids in the treatment of chronic cerebrovascular insufficiency. Curr. Ther. Res. 24(2): 209–226.
31. Ransmayer G, Plörer S, Gerstenbrand F and Bauer G (1987) Double-blind placebo controlled trial of phosphatidylserine in elderly patients with ateriosclerotic encephalopathy. Clin. Trials J. 24: 62–70.
32. Hartmann A (1983) Effect of pentoxifylline on regional cerebral blood flow in patients with cerebral vascular disorders. Eur. Neurol. 22(1): 108–115.
33. Atarashi J, Shoda T, Araki G, Hahora K, Ohyama K and Otano E (1976) Clinical efficacy of pentoxifylline (BL 191) and pyrithioxine hydrochloride in treatment of cerebrovascular disorders. Clin. Eval. 4: 213–230.
34. Buchert D and Hartwart D (1976) Trials of 3,7-dimethyl-1 (5-oxohexyl)xanthine (BL 191) in double blind tests. Farmaco 31: 264–274.
35. Kellner H (1983) Treatment of chronic arterial circulatory disorders: Double-blind trial with pentoxifylline (Trental 400). Pharmacotherapuetica 3(1): 67–73.
36. Harwart D. The treatment of chronic cerebrovascular insufficiency. A double-blind study with pentoxifylline (Trental 400).
37. Hartmann A (1985) Comparative randomized study of cerebral blood flow after long term administration of pentoxifylline and co-dergocrine mesylate in patients with chronic cerebrovascular disease. Curr. Med. Res. Opin. 7: 475–479.
38. Parnetti L, Ciufetti G, Mercuri M, Lupatelli G and Semi U (1986) The role of hemorheological factors in the ageing brain: Long-term therapy with pentoxifylline (Trental 400) in elderly patients with initial mental deterioration. Pharmatherapeutica 10: 617–627.
39. Ghose K (1987) Oxpentifylline in dementia: A controlled study. Arch. Gerontol. Geriat. 6: 19–26.
40. Dominguez D (1986) Vascular dementia and neuropsychological disorders of the ageing brain. In: Gotoh F and Lechner H (eds.) Clinical Hemorheology: A new approach to cerebrovascular disease. Royal Society of Medicine Services. International Congress and Symposium Series No. 100, pp. 14–23.
41. Kazda S, Garthoff B, Krause HP and Schloßmann K (1982) Cerebrovascular effects of the calcium antagonistic dihydropyridine derivate nimodipine in animal experiments. Arzneimittelforsch 32(5): 331–338.
42. Smith ML, Kogsträn E, Rosen I and Siesjö BK (1983) Effect of the calcium antagonist nimodipine on the delayed hypoperfusion following incomplete ischemia in the rat. J. Cereb. Blood Flow Metab. 3: 543–546.

43. Steen PA, Gisvold SE, Milde JH, Newberg LA, Scheithauber BW, Lanner WL and Michenfelder JD (1985) Nimodipine improves outcome when given after complete cerebral ischemia in primates. Anaesthesiology 62: 406–414.
44. Mohammed A (1985) Effect of the calcium antagonist nimodipine on local cerebral blood flow and metabolic coupling. J. Cereb. Blood Flow Metab. 5: 26–33.
45. Meyer FB, Anderson RE, Yaksh TL and Sundt TM (1986) Effect of nimodipine on intracellular brain pH, cortical blood flow, and EEG in experimental focal cerebral ischemia. J. Neurosurg. 64: 617–626.
46. Salgado AV, Jones SC, Furlan AJ, Kortali E, Marshall SA and Little JR (1989) Biomodal treatment with intravenous nimodipine and low-molecular weight dextran for focal cerebral ischemia. Stroke 20: 61.
47. Germano I, Bartkowski H, Nishimura M, Cassel B and Pitts L (1986) The effect of nimodipine in acute experimental cerebral ischemia in the rat. Stroke 17: 144.
48. Fujisawa A, Matsumoto M, Matsuyama T, Neda H, Wanaka A, Yoneda S, Kimura K and Kamada T (1986) The effect of the calcium antagonist nimodipine on the gerbil model of experimental cerebral ischemia. Stroke 17: 748–752.
49. Mabe H, Nagai H, Takagi T, Umemura S and Ohno M (1986) Effect of nimodipine on cerebral functional and metabolic recovery following ischemia in the rat brain. Stroke 17: 501–505.
50. Lazarewicz JW, Pluta R, Salinska E and Puka M (1989) Beneficial effect of nimodipine on metabolic and functional disturbances in rabbit hippocampus following complete cerebral ischemia. Stroke 20: 70–77.
51. Besson JAO, Palin AN, Ebmeier KP, Eagles JM and Smith FN (1988) Calcium antagonists and multi-infarct dementia: A trial involving sequential NMR and psychometric assessment. Int. J. Geriat. Psych. 3: 99–105.
52. Fischhof PK, Wagner G, Littschauer L, Reuther E, Apecechea M (1988) Therapeutic results with nimodipine in primary degenerative dementia and multi-infarct dementia. Workshop Diagnosis and Treatment of Senile Dementia. Seefeld.
53. Dycka J, Schinage N and Volberg E (1986) Placebo-controlled double-blind studies with nimodipine in organic brain syndromes: synopsis of results. In: Bes A, Cahn J, Cahn R, Hoyer S, Marc-Vergnes JP and Wisniewski HM (eds.) Senile Dementias: Early Detection. John Libbey Eurotext, London, Paris, pp. 619–623.
54. Feigenson J, Gitlow H and Greenberg D (1979) The disability oriented stroke unit: A major factor influencing stroke outcome. Stroke 10: 5–8.
55. Smith M, Garraway W, Smith D and Akthar A (1982) Therapy impact on functional outcome in a controlled trial of stroke rehabilitation. Arch. Phys. Med. Rehab. 63: 21–24.
56. Strand T, Asplund K, Eriksson S, Hagg E, Lithner F and Wester P (1985) A non-intensive stroke unit reduces functional disability and the need for long-term hospitalization. Stroke 16: 29–34.
57. Feldman D, Lee P, Unterecker J, Lloyd K, Rusk H and Toole A. (1962) A comparison of functionally oriented medical care and formal rehabilitation in the management of patients with hemiplegia due to cerebrovascular disease. J. Chron. Dis. 15: 297.
58. Waylonis G, Keith N and Aseff J (1973) Stroke rehabilitation in a midwestern country. Arch. Phys. Med. Rehab. 54: 151–155.
59. Peacock P, Riley C, Lampton T, Raffel S and Walker J (1972) The Birmingham stroke epidemiology and rehabilitation study. In: Stewart G (ed.) Trends in Epidemiology: Application to Health Service Research and Training. Springfield Ill: Charles C. Thomas Publisher, pp. 231–346.
60. Wade D, Langton-Hewer R, Wood V, Skilbeck C and Ismail H (1983) The hemiplegic arm after stroke: Measurement and recovery. J. Neurol. Neurosurg. Psychiat. 46: 521–524.
61. Dobkin BH (1989) Focused stroke rehabilitation programs do not improve outcome. Arch. Neurol. 46: 701–703.
62. Reding MJ and McDowell FH (1989) Focused stroke rehabilitation programs improve outcome. Arch. Neurol. 46: 700–701.
63. Robinson RG, Kuhos KL, Starr LB, Roa K and Price TR (1984) Mood disorders in stroke patients. Brain 107: 81–93.

64. Kannel WB, Wolf P and Dawber TR (1978) Hypertension and cardiac impairments increase stroke risk. Geriatrics 33: 71–83.
65. Kannel WB (1971) Current status of the epidemiology of brain infarction associated with occlusion arterial disease. Stroke 2: 295–318.
66. Wolf PA and Kannel WB (1986) Reduction of stroke through risk factors modification. Seminars in Neurology 6: 243–253.
67. Sacco RL, Wolf PA, Kannel WB and McNamara PM (1982) Survival and recurrence following stroke: The Framingham Study. Stroke 13: 3.
68. Friedman GD, Loveland DB, Ehrlich SP (1968) Relationship of stroke to other cardiovascular disease. Circulation 38: 533–541.
69. Wilhelmsen L, Svarsdudd K and Korhan-Bengsten K (1984) Fibrinogen as a risk factor for stroke and myocardial infarction. N. Engl. J. Med. 311: 501–505.
70. Hypertension Detection and Follow-up Program Cooperative Research Group: Five year findings of the hypertension detection and follow-up program: III Reduction in stroke incidence among persons with high blood prerssure. J.A.M.A. 247: 633–638.
71. Mac Mahon SW, Cutler JA, Furberg CD and Payne GH (1986) The effects of drug treatment for hypertension on morbidity and mortality from cardiovascular disease. A review of randomized controlled trials. Prog. Cardiovasc. Dis. 29: 99–118.
72. Whisnant JP (1984) The decline of stroke. Stroke 15: 160–168.
73. Bonita R and Beaglehole R (1989) Increased treatment of hypertension does not explain the decline in stroke mortality in the United States, 1970–1980. Hypertension 13(1): I-69–I-73.
74. Fields WS, Lemak NA, Frankowski RF and Hardy FJ (1977) Controlled trial of aspirin in cerebral ischemia. Stroke 8: 301–316.
75. Canadian Cooperative Study group. A randomized trial of aspirin and dipysidamale in the secondary prevention of atherothrombotic cerebral ischemia. Stroke 14: 45–53.
76. Sorensen PS, Pedersen H, Marquardsen J, Petterson H, Heltberg A, Simonsen N, Munck O and Andersen LA (1983) Acetylsalicylic acid in the prevention of stroke in patients with reversible cerebral ischemic attacks. A Danish cooperative study. Stroke 14: 15–22.
77. A Swedish Cooperative Study (1987) High-dose acetylsalicylic acid after cerebral infarction. Stroke 18: 325–334.
78. Boysen G, Sorensen PS, Juhler M, Andersen AR, Boas J, Olsen JS and Joensen P (1988) Danish very-low-dose aspirin after carotid endarterectomy trial. Stroke 19: 1211–1215.
79. Gent M (1987) Single studies of overview analyses: Is aspirin of value in cerebral ischemia? Stroke 18: 541–544.
80. Bousser MG, Eschwege E, Haguenan M, Lefancconier JM, Thibult N, Touboul D and Touboul PJ (1983) 'AICLA' Controlled trial of aspirin and dipyridamole in the secondary prevention of athero-thrombotic cerebral ischemia. Stroke 14, 5–14.
81. UK-TIA Study Group. United Kingdom transient ischemic attack (UK-TIA) aspirin trial. Br. Med. J. 296: 316–320.
82. The American Canadian Cooperative Study Group: Persantine aspirin trial in cerebral ischemia. Patt II. Endpoint results. Stroke 16: 406–415.
83. European Stroke Prevention Study Group. European stroke prevention study: principal and endpoints. Lancet, December 12, pp. 1351–1354.
84. Matias-Guiu J, Davalos A, Pico M, Monasterio J, Vilasun J and Codina A (1987) Low-dose acetylsalicylic acid (ASA) plus dipyridamole versus dipyridamole alone in the prevention of stroke in patients with reversible ischemic attacks. Acta Neurol. Scand. 76: 413–421.
85. Candeliese L, Landi G, Perrone P, Bracchi M and Brambilla G (1982) A randomized trial of aspirin and sulfinpyrazone in patients with TIA. Stroke 13: 175–179.
86. Sze PC, Reitman D, Pincus MM, Sacks HS and Chalmers TC (1988) Antiplatelet agents in the secondary prevention of stroke: Metaanalysis of the randomized control trials. Stroke 19: 436–442.
87. Antiplatelet trialists collaboration (1988) Secondary prevention of vascular disease by prolonged antiplatelet treatment. Br. Med. J. 296: 320–331.

88. Heyman A, Wilkinson WE, Hurwitz BJ et al. (1984) Risk of ischemic heart disease in patients with TIA. Neurology 34: 626–630.
89. The Canadian Cooperative Study Group. A randomized trial of aspirin and sulfinpyrazone in threatened stroke. N. Engl. J. Med. 299: 53–59.
90. Barnett HJM (1984) Prevention of Stroke. International Anaesthesiology Clinics 22: 11–29.
91. Spranger M, Aspey BSC, Harrison MJG (1989) Sex difference in antithrombotic effect of aspirin. Stroke 20: 34–37.
92. Gent M, Blakeley JA, Easton D et al. The Canadian American ticlopidine study (CATS) in thromboembolic stroke results of a North American randomized trial. N. Engl. J. Med. (in press).
93. The Ticlopidine Aspirin Stroke Study (TASS) Group: The ticlopidine aspirin stroke study (TASS) N. Engl. J. Med. (in press).
94. Lechner H, Ott E, Ossama N and Fazekas F (1986) Follow up studies of the hemorheologic profile in acute ischemic stroke. Clin. Hemorheol. 6: 3–9.
95. Herskovits E, Famulari A, Tamaroff L, Gonzalez AM, Vazquez A, Sund R, Fraiman H, Vila J and Matera V (1981) Randomized trial of pentoxifylline versus acetylsalicylic acid plus dipyridamole in preventing transient ischemic attacks. Lancet 2: 966–968.
96. Herskovits E, Famulari A, Tamaroff L, Gonzalez AM, Vazques A, Dominguez R, Fraiman H and Vila J (1985) Preventive treatment of cerebral transient ischemia: Comparative randomized trial of pentoxifylline versus conventional anti-aggregants. Eur. Neurol. 24: 73–81.
97. Ott E, Körner E and Lechner H (1988) Hemorrheologic treatment of cerebral reversible ischemic episodes with pentoxifylline – a prospective study. Angiology 6: 520–525.
98. Denton E, Barnett HJM, Fields WS, Gent M and Hoak JC (1977) Cerebral Ischemia: The role of thrombosis and antithrombotic therapy. Study Group of antithrombotic therapy. Stroke 8: 150–175.
99. Lodder J, Dennis MS, Raak L van, Jones LN and Warlow CP (1988) Cooperative study on the value of long term anti-coagulation in patients with stroke and non-rheumatic artrial fibrillation. Br. Med. J. 296: 1435–1438.
100. Gustaffson C and Britton M (1986) Prognosis after brain infarction in patients with non-rheumatica-trial fibrillation compared with sinus rhythm. Acta. Neurol. Scand. 73: 520–521.
101. Norrving B, Nilsson B and Risberg J (1982) rCBF in patients with carotid occlusion: Resting and hypercapnic flow related to collateral pattern. Stroke 13: 155–162.
102. Forfar JC (1979) A seven year analysis of hemorrhage in patients on long term anticoagulant treatment. Br. Heart J. 42: 128–132.
103. Wolf PA, Dawber TR, Thomas HE et al. (1983) Epidemiologic assessment of chronic atrial fibrillation and risk of stroke. The Framingham study. Stroke 14: 664–667.
104. Pessin MS, Duncan GW, Mohr JP and Poskanzer DC (1977) Clinical and angiographic features of carotid transient ischemic attacks. N. Engl. J. Med. 296: 358–362.
105. Levin S, Sondheimer F and Levin J (1980) The contralateral diseased but asymptomatic carotid artery: To operate or not? An update. Am. J. Surg. 140: 203–205.
106. Wolf PA, Kannel WB, Sorlie P and McNamara P (1981) Asymptomatic carotid bruit and risk of stroke. J.A.M.A. 245: 1442–1445.
107. Heyman A, Wilkinson W, Heyden et al. (1980) Risk of stroke in asymptomatic persons with cervical arterial bruits: A population study in Evans county Georgia. N. Engl. J. Med. 302: 838–841.
108. Busutill RW, Baker JD, Davidson RK and Machleder HI (1981) Carotid artery stenosis-hemodynamic significance and clinical course. J.A.M.A. 245: 1438–1441.
109. Eastcott HG, Pickering GW and Robb C (1954) Reconstruction of internal carotid artery in a patient with intermittent hemiplegia. Lancet 2: 994–996.
110. Thompson JE and Garett WV (1980) Peripheral arterial surgery. N. Engl. J. Med. 302: 491–503.
111. Thompson JE (1982) Controversies in carotid surgery. Arch. Surg. 117: 1072.
112. The EC/IC Bypass Study Group. Failure of extracranial-intracranial arterial bypass to reduce the risk of ischemic stroke. N. Engl. J. Med. 313: 1191–1200.
113. Millikan CH (1985) Treatment of occlusive cerebrovascular disease. Cerebrovascular Survey Report of the National Institute of Neurological and Communicative Disorders and Stroke.

114. Norrving B and Nilsson B (1986) Cerebral embolism of cardiac origin, the limited possibilities of secondary prevention. Acta Neurol. Scand. 73: 520.
115. Yonekura M, Austin G and Hayward W (1982) Long-term evaluation of cerebral blood flow, transient ischemic attacks and stroke after STA-MCA anastomosis. Surg. Neurol. 18: 123–130.
116. Baron JC, Bousser MG, Rey A, Guillard A, Ocomar D and Castoigne P (1981) Reversal of focal 'misery perfusion' syndrome by extra-intracranial arterial bypass in hemodynamic cerebral ischemia: A case study with 150 positron emission tomography. Stroke 12: 454–459.
117. Cote R and Caron JL (1988) Management of carotid artery occlusion. Stroke 23: 25–29.
118. Relman AS (1987) The extracranial-intracranial arterial bypass study. What have we learned? N. Engl. J. Med. 316: 809–810.
119. Sundt TM (1987) Was the international randomized trial of extracranial intracranial arterial bypass representative of the population at risk. N. Engl. J. Med. 316: 814–816.
120. Barnett HJM, Sackett D, Taylor DW et al. (1987) Are the results of the extracranial/intracranial bypass trial generalizable? N. Engl. J. Med. 316: 820–824.
121. Dyken ML and Pokras R (1984) The performance of endarterectomy for disease of the extracranial arteries of the head. Stroke 15: 948–955.
122. Warlow C (1984) Carotid endarterectomy: Does it work? Stroke 15: 1068–1080.
123. Fields WS, Maslenikov V, Meyer JS, Hass WK, Remington RD and Macdonald M (1970) Joint study of extracranial occlusion. J.A.M.A. 211: 1993–2003.
124. Shaw DA, Venables GS, Cartlidge NEF, Bates D and Dickinson PIT (1984) Carotid endarterectomy in patients with transient cerebral ischemia. J. Neurol. Sci. 64: 45–53.
125. Jonas S (1986) IMPS (intact months of patient survival) an analysis of the results of carotid endarterectomy. Stroke 17: 1329–1336.
126. Whisnant JP, Sandok BA and Sundt TM (1963) Carotid endarterectomy for unilateral carotid system transient cerebral ischemia. Mayo Clin. Proc. 58: 171–175.
127. Takolander RJ, Bergenti SE and Ericson BF (1983) Carotid artery surgery in patients with minor stroke. Br. J. Surg. 70: 13–16.
128. Erikson SE, Link H, Alm A, Radberg C and Kostulas V (1981) Results from 88 consecutive prophylacitic carotid endarterectomy in cerebral infarcts and transitory ischemic attacks. Acta Neurol. Scand. 63: 209–219.
129. Cantelmo NL, Cutler BS, Whecker HB, Herrmann JB and Cardullo PA (1981) Early detection of carotid stenosis following endarterectomy. Arch. Surg. 116: 1005–1008.
130. Kremen JE, Gee W, Kaupp HA and McDonald KM (1979) Restenosis or occlusion after carotid endarterectomy. Arch. Surg. 114: 608–610.
131. Nicholls SC, Phillips DJ, Bergelin RO, Beach KW, Primozich JF and Strandness E (1985) Carotid endarterectomy. Relationship of the outcome to early restenosis. J. Vasc. Surg. 2: 375–381.
132. Taylor DW, Sackett DL and Haynes RB (1984) Sample size for randomized trials in stroke prevention. How many patients do we need? Stroke 15: 968–971.
133. North American Symptomatic Carotid Endarterectomy Study Group. Carotid endarterectomy: Three critical evaluations. Stroke 18: 987–989.
134. Agnoli A (1986) Nimodipine in chronic cerebrovascular disease. Proceedings 4th European Workshop on Clinical Neuropharmacology. Calcium Antagonists and Cerebral Ischemia. Pamplona, p. 36.
135. Cosni F, Caresia L and Panebianco G (1986) Treatment of chronic cerebrovascular insufficiency: Comparison between nimodipine and dihydroergotoxine. Clin. Ther. (Rome) 116(3): 213–220.
136. Dorn M (1984) Therapie der zerebrovaskulären Insuffizienz mit Nimodipin. Psycho 10(3): 186–196.
137. Held K, Boehme K, Rode CP (1985) Efficacy and Tolerability of nimodipine in patients with old age cerebrovascular dysfunction. In: Nimodipine: Pharmacological and Clinical Properties (Betz E, Deck K, Hoffmeister F, eds.) Schattauer Verlag, Stuttgart, New York, pp. 289–293.
138. Maio di L, Campanella G, Somma di S, Divitiis de O, Gagliosdi R, Caresia L (1987) Nimodipine: A new drug for the treatment of organic brain syndromes. Acta Therapeutica 13: 61–70.

Part Three

Concluding Comments

Concluding comments

Helmut Lechner
Department of Neurology and Psychiatry, Karl-Franzens University, Graz, Austria

Cerebrovascular disease in its acute form, a stroke, still remains a major threat not only to the ageing population but also to younger persons. Although there has been a marked decrease in mortality in some western countries during the last thirty years, a noticeable rise in the death-rates can still be observed in developing countries. Despite the fact that stroke has become the third most common cause of death and disability (after heart disease and cancer), there exists a remarkably low awareness among the general public of the potentially fatal consequences for the patient and of the huge burden for both society and the family.

The various pathophysiological mechanisms leading to acute or chronic cerebrovascular disease have been broadly discussed. They include sudden cerebral occlusions due to thrombosis or embolism, the role of haemorrheological factors, various mechanisms generating platelet aggregation and adhesion as well as endothelial damage, cellular destruction by free radicals or intercellular calcium overload. Under ischaemic conditions secondary metabolic processes lead to the accumulation of lactate with vasoparalysis and damage in deeper compartments, and furthermore to the development of cytotoxic and vasogenic brain oedema. Therapeutic measures should be aimed at protecting the neurons in the penumbra and at maintaining cerebral function.

The development of new non-invasive diagnostic techniques provided high-quality imaging of the location of ischaemic lesions, information on regional and global cerebral blood flow as well as on the cerebral metabolic rate of oxygen and on the status of cerebral arteries. Thus, the regional cerebral states, including morphology and function, can reliably indicate the appropriate therapeutic measures.

The clinical picture of acute cerebral ischaemic events depends on the location of the affected area, and the classification also includes the duration of clinical symptoms. Differentiation is made between TIA, RIND, completed stroke and multi-infarct dementia, where the anatomical background is constituted by multiple infarctions, lacunae and watershed lesions.

The management of acute ischaemic strokes should consider an appropriate haemodilution and thrombolysis, the use of haemorheological agents and of calcium channel blockers. Newer studies on the value of 21-amino-steroids and of superoxide dismutase in reducing the damaging effects of free radicals offer optimism for future therapies in patients with acute ischaemic stroke.

The chronic forms of cerebrovascular disease such as vascular dementia present an increasing problem in our ageing society and are subject to extensive experimental and clinical research. Clinical assessment remains the mainstay and most reliable method for determining multi-infarct dementia.

Hachinski's ischaemic score is reliable in distinguishing MID from Alzheimer's disease but unable to discriminate between MID and mixed dementia. For a therapeutic approach, however, this seems to be irrelevant since the identification of a vascular component is potentially subject to treatment and prevention. However, there exists a strong need for a redefinition of vascular dementia, as patients with vascular ischaemic components are statistically underestimated.

The design of clinical trials is an essential prerequisite to establishing an adequate treatment of MID. The use of the modified Hachinski Score, the Mini Mental Status Examination and the Alzheimer Disease Assessment Scale present an efficient clinical model as realised in a controlled trial with pentoxifylline.

In summary, the treatment of chronic cerebrovascular disease is directed, on the one hand, towards the prevention of recurrent ischaemic events, and on the other hand, towards the improvement of cognitive function as well as of the concomitant symptoms – and thus, of the patient's quality of life.

The control of risk factors for acute and chronic cerebrovascular disease is of crucial importance for both the improvement of quality of life and for secondary prevention. Arterial hypertension, cardiac disease, diabetes and smoking habits are the major predictive factors for ischaemic stroke. Appropriate control and management of these factors may decrease morbidity and mortality due to cerebrovascular disease.

It is therefore an essential goal to identify at least those 10% of the asymptomatic population in which 50% of all strokes will occur, as the Framingham study suggests. It is likewise as important to detect and treat the high-risk TIA group as it is mandatory to closely monitor patients with cardiac and peripheral vascular disease for their cerebrovascular status.

Whilst stroke is the most severe manifestation of acute cerebrovascular disease, the chronic forms remain a major medical and socioeconomic problem. Our goal is therefore to establish progress in cerebrovascular disease by enhancing our efforts in clinical research in order to achieve the most efficient therapeutic measures possible. This goal, however, can only be reached if we succeed in creating a high level of awareness concerning the devastating status of patients with stroke and vascular dementia – similar to the attention with which Alzheimer's disease and its consequences have been received.

Index of authors